What People Are Saying

Nine's a Charm

Martha Gray's Pagan Portals book, *Nine's a Charm: Herbs of the Anglo-Saxon Healing Poem*, is a beautifully crafted, insightful book about this often overlooked aspect of Anglo-Saxon magic. Written with clear expertise and herbal experience, Martha's writing is concise and engaging, which makes her the perfect teacher to guide you along this seldom-explored herbal path. Each of the nine herbs is explored meticulously, including rigorously researched folklore, Anglo-Saxon and Norse archaeological evidence, mythic exploration (including various connections to the gods), growing guides, and historical to modern medicinal usage. As a Galdor practitioner myself, I was intrigued to read Martha's informative instruction on this magical craft in relation to the Nine Herbs Charm — something I had not ever considered. Additionally, the recipes are very welcome — I enjoyed the Chervil and Carrot Soup! Martha Gray's book is sure to be a well-thumbed favourite on many bookshelves. It will certainly be on mine.

Thea Prothero, author of *A Guide to Pilgrimage*

At first glance, the Anglo-Saxon Nine Herb Charm is just a simple poem. But Martha Gray's book *Nine's a Charm* explores the great depths of the verses and the herbs within them, from both magical and medicinal perspectives, showing that there's far more here than first meets the eye. Complemented by a foreword by Shani Oates that puts the charm in historical perspective, this book is a fascinating journey into history, magic, and herbalism that's sure to interest a wide variety of readers.

Laura Perry, founder and Temple Mom of Ariadne's Tribe and author of *Pantheon - The Minoans*

Pagan Portals
Nine's a Charm

Herbs of the Anglo-Saxon Healing Poem

Pagan Portals
Nine's a Charm

Herbs of the Anglo-Saxon Healing Poem

Martha Gray

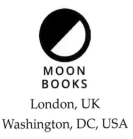

MOON BOOKS

London, UK
Washington, DC, USA

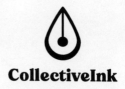

CollectiveInk

First published by Moon Books, 2025
Moon Books is an imprint of Collective Ink Ltd.,
Unit 11, Shepperton House, 89 Shepperton Road, London, N1 3DF
office@collectiveinkbooks.com
www.collectiveinkbooks.com
www.moon-books.net

For distributor details and how to order please visit the 'Ordering' section on our website.

Text copyright: Martha Gray 2024

ISBN: 978 1 80341 456 0
978 1 80341 457 7 (ebook)
Library of Congress Control Number: 2024935724

All rights reserved. Except for brief quotations in critical articles or reviews, no part of this book may be reproduced in any manner without prior written permission from the publishers.

The rights of Martha Gray as author have been asserted in accordance with the Copyright, Designs and Patents Act 1988.

A CIP catalogue record for this book is available from the British Library.

Design: Lapiz Digital Services

UK: Printed and bound by CPI Group (UK) Ltd, Croydon, CR0 4YY
US: Printed and bound by Thomson-Shore, 7300 West Joy Road, Dexter, MI 48130

We operate a distinctive and ethical publishing philosophy in all areas of our business, from our global network of authors to production and worldwide distribution.

Contents

Foreword	xi
Introduction – The Healing Charm	1
Chapter 1 – Mugwart (Mugwort)	11
Chapter 2 – Waybread (Plantain)	18
Chapter 3 – Stune (Watercress)	23
Chapter 4 – Stithe / Venom-loathe (Betony)	28
Chapter 5 – Chamomile	33
Chapter 6 – Wergulu (Nettle)	42
Chapter 7 – Apple (Crab Apple)	52
Chapter 8 – Fennel	69
Chapter 9 – Fille (Chervil)	77
Chapter 10 – Thyme	92
Conclusion	101
Bibliography	102

This book is dedicated to Suzanne Ruthven who passed away suddenly on 1ˢᵗ January 2024. She was a great inspiration to me and may she continue to inspire others through her works.

I also dedicate this book to my husband, Chris, who has given me encouragement and support during the writing of this work. It has meant more to me than he will ever know.

Abbreviations

OE – Old English

Foreword

"Lef mon læces behofað"
(A sick man needs a leech) [1]

As an independent scholar of the magics and beliefs of the medieval world, I have a vested interest in the charming and mythic traditions of northern peoples. It is therefore my privilege to compose an introduction for this book written to shine a light on one of the most enigmatic yet revealing charms of the Anglo-Saxon world.[2] Straggling the modalities of herb-lore, magic and culture, *The Lay of the Nine Herbs Charm* is a wonderful exposition on early medieval life. Being hael and hearty in this era was an impossible challenge, even for the most-hardy of folk. Death and disease were constant companions. Any skill that could help to combat this sense of impending doom was embraced wholeheartedly, and clung to somewhat tenaciously, despite adversities in socio-religious politicking. It was largely the work of specialists, though the non-specialist undoubtedly dabbled too. *The Lay of the Nine Herbs* is used by the author to command a base-line for exploration into the noble craft of herbalism, through a range of applications for the modern practitioner seeking deeper knowledge of their craft. The work undertaken here by the present author encompasses medicinal, magical and culinary uses for the nine glorious herbs featured in this famous charm.

'Cræft' is a word once used by the Anglo-Saxons for the concoction of a medical prescription which relied very much upon the capture of the plant's vital essence. Signifying power and knowledge, or 'virtue, it was the primary aim of the leech to obtain as much 'cræft' as possible, to enable all disease to overcome or supress the invasion of hostile forces upon body and mind. Despite the wry attitude in relation to the medieval 'leech', combating the visible and the invisible facets of nature was a challenging and disciplined undertaking. When studying the few Saxon herbals that have survived (albeit as scribal copies in manuscript form), we are hard pressed to remember they are sourced in yet older manuscripts that certainly perished during the interminable Danish invasions. Beyond this, the oldest bound script we possess is from the 10th century.

Our knowledge of Anglo-Saxon plant lore is therefore found almost exclusively in the four primary sources: the *Leech Book of Bald*, the *Lácnung* (as named by Cockayne) the so-called Περὶ Διδαξέων, and the Saxon translation of the 4th century '*Herbarium*,' (*Herbarium Apuleii Platonici*, also known as Pseudo-Apuleius) whose author desired association with Apuleius of Madaura (124–170 C.E.), the Roman poet and philosopher. Modern scholars no longer uphold this attribution. As an original work, the *Lácnung* (Harl. 585), is one of the oldest and most interesting manuscripts. Unlike some other works, this small, thick volume is without illustrations, although some of the letters are illuminated and somewhat crudely ornamented. Nearly all the amuletic and remedial charms not found within the *Leech Book of Bald*, feature in the (Northumbrian) Harley 585 (late 11th century) and in Harley 6258 b (12th century). Both manuscripts are now housed in the British Museum.

Studies of these texts show that Anglo Saxon herblore and medical knowledge was largely elementary, yet quite wide-ranging. Many herbs were known of, but only a handful were properly understood and could be found in popular use, albeit repeated many times in quite rudimentary formulas. Cures depended upon folk medicines gleaned from vernacular translations of those former Graeco-Roman works, including prayers and quasi-magical procedures, some of which contain phrases of doggerel Latin. Magic and medicine of this early medieval period is based is the classical works of Pliny,

Dioscorides and of Marcellus Empiricus; for instance, we know that Bede was very familiar with the works of Hippocrates. The Anglo-Saxons themselves did not contribute any new observations relating to plant-lore, not even of native plants, until approximately 1120 C.E., as evidenced within *De material medica*, and the *Herbarius*. As a result, most of the plants cited were unknown to the physicians using them in England for treatments and remedies. Because even simple terms initially derive from Latin, any attempt to distinguish plant names of English origin within these pharmacopoeias is almost futile. In the absence of the (later) standard classification system (ie. *Linnaean*), errors of identification and analysis compounded yet further the scribal errors accrued when copying those early manuscripts. Several plant names belonging to the medieval pharmacopoeia are similar, creating confusions whereby clarity was lost; many plant names are now lost to time.

Any practical knowledge of medicine and surgery known to the ancient Britons was probably absorbed by the peoples who settled in these Isles after the departure of the Romans in the 5th century. The Teutonic peoples brought with them some provincial knowledge of the properties of worts, which they freely employed, and although their empirical knowledge of herbs was in many cases intermixed with a certain amount of superstition in the form of charms and incantations, this formed the basis of the medical art practised by the Anglo-Saxons in England. Perched upon the cusp of transition and change, medicine during the early medieval period – as recorded in the *Lácnung* – blended together a wide range of medicine along with continental folk magics. Rapid conversion began soon after their arrival, settling over native beliefs and practises of an animistic nature. They quickly began to develop a literature of their own that continued to involve the northern runes, but now incorporated a new alphabet, parchment, and ink. Thus were the foundations of Anglo-Saxon culture reforged.

Enriched through the Christian missions of the Graeco-Roman world tradition, both directly and through trade, early Anglo-Saxon[3] medicine and herb-cræft thus relied heavily upon an inherited knowledge of classical pharmacopoeia – consisting of plants whose origins were Mediterranean – and various plants of European origin. As noted above, very few were native species, despite the names given to them in translation for their own compilations. Nonetheless, superstition prevailed in their idiosyncratic construction and application; the seemingly irrational practice of magic was invoked more often than not.

Interpolations of (Teutonic) folk-lore made to the Latin classical texts garnered from eastern (Eurasian), Ecclesiastical treatises, merged to create a unique foundation in the four humours, elements, solar way markers. This blended perfectly with the Teutonic obsession concerning the four cardinal points (that are also a significant feature in Finnish shamanic healing rituals). Classical medicine and indeed its philosophy resided in the dynamic between the micro-macrocosmic worlds, which again merged seamlessly into the mythic world view of the Anglo-Saxon who saw everything as a reflection of the 'otherworld.' Their cosmology was simple, it comprised only of the seen and the unseen. Physiology was intrinsically linked to cosmology. Health and well-being was a celestial and terrestrial matter.

From letters written to Boniface, the Apostle of the Germans, by correspondents in England, it would appear that medical literature did exist here as early as the 8th century, since in one letter, we find his comment: *"We have some medical books, but the foreign ingredients we find prescribed in them are unknown to us, and difficult to obtain."* However, there were no professional treatises nor famous, named physicians, merely notebooks from reputable 'leeches.' Læca (leche) is the Anglo-Saxon word for physician, with lácnung meaning a remedy or medicine proscribed by them. Information is quite rudimentary, dealing mainly with broken bones, sickness, abrasions, headaches and inflammations. Moreover, the internal mechanics of the body baffled them, and everything was seen as 'invasion' or attack from invisible spirits whose 'elf-shot' was the cause of illness and festering wounds. They had no understanding of endemic disease, and epidemics utterly confounded them. The few works we have are testament to this. The existence of the professional leech (be he layman or ecclesiastical) is noted in the 7th century laws of king Æthelberht of Kent.

Charms and charming are terms used widely and commonly applied, often without attention to critical nuances of intent, or even of consideration to their appropriateness. Because we often inherit words in a cavalier fashion, I would like to take a moment to explore the actual meanings of these terms, a brief deviation that I hope will facilitate a better grasp of what worts and wort-cunning is really about. The etymology of the word 'charm' perfectly encapsulates the performative aspect of those early texts, and engages with the Anglo-Saxon term – *galdor*, which appears in diverse texts glossed (for *incantata*). These appear in homilies, psalms and biblical translations when referring to witchcraft, spells and enchantments. While 'charm' does bear superstitious connotations relating to the supernatural, alternatives such as spell or incantation, share little of those nuances, and enforce only vague semantics. The term 'charm' is therefore unsatisfactory, but must suffice in lieu of suitable alternatives.

A charm may therefore be considered as a performative text having ritualistic activity and archaic elements that engage the 'Other.' This definition does not therefore exclude the Christian texts, those that relate, for instance, to prayers or the various Masses, which to all extents and purposes, are magical formulae, spoken or sung, and are arguably indistinct from heathen charms utilising galdor. Some might argue that (Heathen) charms do not make their appeals directly and explicitly to 'God' for his assistance, or that prayers are generally constructed as a mode of communication with God. I would counter that quite baldly, stating that this is an under sight that miscalculates the depth of the unwritten (and unspoken) acknowledgment of the 'Other'. In terms of qualitive content, expectancy of outcome and intent, I see little difference between them, and for this reason, a better appreciation of the charms is discovered whereby they may be approached on their own terms, without pre-conception or need to categorise them as Heathen or Christian, either partially or wholly. This did not matter to our ancestors, and it should not matter to us. Ultimately, efficacy depends upon sincerity, integrity and a sound knowledge of herb craft. The author of this book supplies all this and more.

Anglo-Saxon charms mainly deal with mundane issues relating to stolen cattle, goods, health of cattle and people. Several charms employ mood-enhancing techniques achieved through sympathetic narratives that effectively set the stage (and precedent) for the work ahead. The re-creation of a given situation will generate the requisite correspondence and secure the 'virtue' needed to bring the charm to fruition. Among the earliest charms, short but succinct narratives relate epic deeds of curative superiority that work to dispel the invasive disease spirit by intimidation and diminishment. Nine is a number generally found in popular diminishing charms, generally for warts, and was sacred to both Heathen and Catholic alike. Mental illness was considered to be a sure sign of possession. Followers of Hippocrates consider maleness in association with the right side of the body, and femaleness with the left. Three is sacred to Roman deities, nine to those deemed to be 'Celtic,' (possibly Catholic aligned with Catholic influences), manifest in the rosary, the Mass, and as a sacred novena. Three and nine are also sacred to the Finnish peoples. This dynamic connection between an epic precedent and the desired result is evident in the Merseburg liberation charm. Success was meted by analogy.

In similar manner, despite the reference to Christ (as the holy lord in heaven and as he who stood over the venom), Woden is named as the heroic exorcist able to vanquish malefica in *The Lay of the Nine Herbs*. Charms with narrative (heroic) passages occur in almost all Indo-European languages, and even in Celtic, Slavonic, and Greco-Italic tongues. In the Ugrian group of languages, the magic songs of the Finns present many interesting examples of spells containing similar characteristics. All magical and ritual specialists will invariably call upon names and forms most familiar to them culturally, even if adaptations and addendums cite or list those of others. *The Nine Herbs Charm* is a prime example of this. The cumulative construct of such charms in whatever form they are found in, or adapted to, was simply a matter of practicality.

Spanning several centuries from the cusp of the so-called 'Dark Ages' in the 5th century to the Norman invasion of the 11th century, the Anglo-Saxon world was complex and ever shifting. In that time, the world opened up, trade and movement introduced innovations in farming, animal husbandry, crafts and arts, but I think the biggest impact was on belief. In turn, this influenced the approach to magic and medicine as creative enterprises aligned to the natural and supernatural worlds. Folklore and folk medicine are inexorably linked, such that belief permeates every aspect of life, ranging from the wonders of creation to the terror and fear of death and beyond. The time spent in-between was therefore determined by, and dependent upon, health and survival; this required knowledge and understanding, daring and dedication. This was an era when legends (meaning, what is *read*, as opposed to what is spoken in oral tradition) were generated in abundance. Miraculous deeds were recorded as much for the purpose of performative expression (edification rather than entertainment) as much as they were for posterity.

The Early Medieval period was literally plagued with a series of epidemics, yet the Anglo-Saxon sources are silent on this grave matter. Between the 6th-8th centuries especially, the devastation was wide-spread, and no doubt contributed to the escalating fear promoted by the Church that these were demonic visitations for unrequited sins. Hunger and pestilence increased the fevered desperation for atonement. Famine and infestation[4] took its toll on mind and body, as each broke down beneath its inimitable force. Cattle too as the main source of income and food security, were devasted. Bede gives account of the flux that raged from Kent to Northumbria in 664 C.E., causing the East Saxons to turn to idolatry, before being shown the error of their ways. Alongside the fear-mongering of the Church, this is the context for the composition and application of *The Lay of the Nine Herbs*. To properly understand the latter, we must properly appreciate the impact of the former. Preparation of the herbs in this charm asks for certain words to be sung the over them at various stages: three times before brewing, and then upon the apple likewise; and again, before the salve is applied. A directive is given to sing the charm into the patient's mouth and into both his ears and into the wound. Singing into the ear apparently frightens the spirit possessing the body, a ruse utilised to great effect by the AS exorcist.[5]

In the majority of English spells, the evil spirit is not directly referred to. Yet even in these cases, it is easy to conclude from the remedies prescribed, that malevolent, superhuman beings are regarded as the agents of all varieties of illnesses. Diseases attributed to devils and demons (which included Heathen land and ancestral spirits) by the Church, largely remained perceived of as elves by Anglo-Saxon peoples, despite the actuation of considerable levels of conversion (in England) during the 6th century. Such levels of conversion did not reach Scandinavia until the 10th century, although Sweden began conversion as early as the 8th century. Pestilence and disease were rife and began to take form as perceived monsters, as beasts of torment and affliction. Relief from such grievous ordeals came through 'god's grace' in the form of fiery bolts from heaven, a concept that may have influenced the description of Woden's glory twigs. In fact, the passage relating to mugwort – *"She is strong against the onflight, She is strong against those evil things that fare throughout the land"*[6] – in *The Lay of the Nine Herbs* (found in the *Lácnung LXXIX*) very much reflects this notion of disease as a monstrous form. What is particularly interesting is that the colours associated with each venom reflect various disorders: of the blood (red), bile (yellow), skin (green), bowel (brown or black), organs (purple), mind and mental issues (blue), breath and respiratory system (white). These correspondences appear to have some correlation with the twigs used by Woden in this special charm. Colour vocabulary was of unique importance to the Saxons, a trait not much explored within classical medicine. Red plants were deemed efficacious for men, green for women.

Appeals to the 'Other' were made through prayer and propitiation. Deliverance from epidemics was eventually cited as the work of saints whose intervention and sacrifice were explained as god's grace. In other words, healing did not transpire through human hand. Superstition prevailed during this severely challenging time, making pragmatism a rare trait. Various chronicles record accounts of sightings of grim omens in the skies, of extreme weather anomalies that included whirlwinds, lightning and even of fiery dragons. It is not insignificant that the etymology of Gullveig means hurricane (violent storm)! The terror of disease and famine were exacerbated by a sudden (interstitial) cold snap towards the end of the 7th century, which fuelled fears that accrued to the extent that when the Danish invasion began 100 years later, it was seen as just punishment for sin – whence it was hailed as god's wrath. Invasion of self and of land were indistinguishable features of Anglo-Saxon disease. Both were fought on the same terms. Continual warring against the invasions exacerbated the devastation to land, cattle and human life. These were troubling times on a scale we cannot begin to imagine.

What is particularly interesting is the distinguishing references found in *Olaf's Saga* (chp. 247) to women nurses in attendance at the Battle of Stiklestad in 1030 C.E., and to leeches, whom we must therefore presume were men. Sources are silent on the existence of female leeches. Support for this exclusivity occurs in the comments relating to the (male) leeches who attended King Magnus the Good, two of whom were Icelanders, who were thereafter known as the greatest of leeches, from whom it is claimed that all leeches were descended. Herbal salves of wine, oil, honey and comfrey were common in the treatment for wounds incurred on the battlefield. It is an odd fact that more Anglo-Saxon kings died in battle than in their beds. Life was harsh unyielding, punishing. It was never less than uncompromising.

According to an old AS herbal, Lady's Day (Feast of the Annunciation) was traditionally the time for the return to order after the upheaval and chaos of the winter storms, and of death, health, poverty, hunger etc. Lady's day appropriately announces the official year because of this. It carries the potency and promise of the fecund, quickening tide. Chaos is supressed through the imposition of order. Reflecting this marvel of Nature, a medieval herbalist maintained that the leafage (of a plant) heals from the Annunciation (March 25th) to The Feast of St. Peter and St. Paul (June 29th), the stalk from the Nativity of St. John the Baptist (June 24th) to Michaelmas (Sept 29th); root from the Epiphany to Spring, cycling us back to the Annunciation again.[7]

Almost every month in the year is prescribed in Anglo-Saxon recipes as the prime time for gathering certain herbs. The numbers in each month increase as the summer advances and decrease as we approach winter. According to Pliny,

Midsummer was especially potent. Mugwort is cited as very potent when picked at this time, especially at noon. Grimm gives various examples of herbs to be gathered at this time. One of them, *Walpurgiskraut*, blooms exactly at midnight on St John's Eve, and the picking of it is attended by storm and thunder; but whoever gets possession of it becomes rich and able to prophesy. Midsummer Day is devoted to all forms of exorcism.[8] Pennies were commonly used as weights to measure herbal prescriptions. Time (for steeping or cooking) was measured in the number of psalms or other prayers were repeated.

Many herbs were deemed especially potent if gathered on festival days: everlasting (*Gnaphalium*) on Ascension Day as a charm against lightning, and in ancient Wales, pennyroyal on Whit-Sunday or the eve of St. John the Baptist, for the benefit of a person who has lost consciousness or speech, in consequence of illness. Besides the season or feast-day of the week, (Friday was deemed to be auspicious), the hour too is important.[9] Hours for gathering at optimum potency was sunrise, or noon. Mandrake and sea holly should be culled under the moon, after sunset, or, before sunrise – either, with dew still upon them. The baneful moon is the legacy of the classical herbalists, Pliny noted that all vegetables should be cut while the moon wanes rather than waxing. Lucan especially was of the opinion that the Moon (summoned by malignant forces) shed its baneful influence upon all herbs if cut when its light fell upon them. He advised they should be gathered only when the moon waned. Ovid advocated the gathering should be preferably undertaken with bronze or copper scythes. Anglo-Saxons preferred short wands of ivory (antler) or iron (where specified in the charms only). Numerous rites and rituals have been developed over hundreds of years for the most beneficent gathering of herbs for magical or medicinal use. In certain cases, taboos are in full force to ensure the optimum cautions are in place and that efficacy was maximised.

Iron must not be used on betony, mandrake, waybread and burdock, but was promoted for gathering sea-holly (the gatherer must also avert their gaze from the toxic influences of the 'creatures that wrap around the latter's roots. To prevent this influence 'bleeding' out to other plants near to it, circles must be drawn around the rooted area (using iron), while glancing westwards, away from the plant. (Mandrake too). Plants were always pulled in silence using the left (female) hand, in fact, silence was generally advocated, though enchantments could be sung (softly), repetitions of prayers for example, and statements of intent relating primarily to the intended use. Mugwort especially like to be informed of its purpose. Whereas the Teutonic mind recognised the plant spirit present in the herbs, the Christian thought this blasphemous, being of the mind that Christ healed through them, having no 'virtue,' of their own. Hence their usage was directed under the blessings of genuflection. This precaution was similarly extended to all food stuffs and beverages.

We do not know for certain what actual form early Heathen charms took, as those that remain in the records are an admixture of all concurrent influences, wherein attributions to any form of spirit is substituted with that of Christ, whether Finnish or Teutonic. It is now generally accepted that of all the charms, the only ones deemed to be purely Heathen, are the two Merseburg charms. It is highly probable that the tradition they sprang from heavily influenced *The Lay of the Nine Herbs Charm*. Conversion was a continual battle of minds and souls, an issue the Church was forced to adopt certain compromising strategies in, at least initially. Sacred places were absorbed where possible and destroyed if not. Altars and relics replaced the rough *hörgr* (Old Norse, pl. *hörgar*) or *hearg*, and *stelae* of the heathen cultic landscape. Pope Gregory believed that a slow siege would better secure stable converts.

Generally, we can say that substitutions for names were the order of the day. We have lost so many local (spirit) forms, whose names were relevant only to a select few people in any given region. Saints replaced many of these, and so we may never know who they were originally. Classes of spirits have added to the confusion. Holden and Perchten were originally described as 'troops' of demons, without individuality or singular identity. It is ironic that the Church in its zealous drive to diminish the potency of local heathen spirits, should have personified these troops into (female) leaders, known as Holda (Hulda) and Perchta,[10] while affording them greater importance than Freyja. Wodan (Woden) is another good example of this erroneous elevation, so it is entirely possible that like the holden and perchten, he was also a descriptor for a class of wild spirit. His fame and import then grew (beyond the region where his status was already significant) through 'legend' ascribed to him.

Although many later myths demonstrate obvious signs of fusion (that of Baldur's fate is a prime example), the native wights of hearth and home were harder to eradicate, and many of these were called upon in the surviving charming traditions of the Anglo Saxon and Danish peoples. The names we are now accustomed to hearing in modern popular traditions, such as Óðinn and Þör, are almost silent in the records and chronicles of all Heathen peoples (except where their condemnation is referred to in Christian texts). Þör is sometimes found inscribed on amulets, and in only a handful of the (later) written charming traditions that remain to us. The eradication of all magical, ritualistic practises namely *Wiccecræft fyrht,* was of much greater concern to the Church, taking precedence over lingering beliefs in elemental spirits. The belief in 'monsters' of alleged super-human strength (Grendel for example), who lived in Mountainous caves, bogs and sink holes below water, were part of the cultural influences of the Angles and peoples of Norway and Finland, where Trolls, giants, elves and dwarves were commonplace. The Teuton shared much with the Finn regarding the spirits of land and water.

We have no precise translations of the correct meanings of Anglo-Saxon terms used to describe all things 'Other', and our estimations fall short of the nuances of the originals. Amongst these we may include the AS *galdor* (Old High German – *galdar*), meaning incantation, that has its origins in words relating to singing. A similar Old Norse term is *galdor*, also meaning a (singing) charm; This differs from the spell which is spoken; Spilla is found in the Gothic bible where it is used to describe 'old wives fables.' In other words, a spell bears a sense of the fabulous, and of a narrative tradition. Singing is another strong Finnish tradition. The Kalevala is replete with magical songs and fables. As cultural examples of socio-religiosity, all stories, poems[11] and charms are as important as the magics they preserve within them. Of course, Óðinn is later credited with being the master of Skald-cræft. His rune-cræft was condemned as wizardry, just as the Ás-folk he represented, were known as 'wizard' smiths.

The cutting, carving, (blooding), naming and use of runic staves is attested since pre-Christian times. Tán (lot) is a twig, *wuldertánas* is interpreted as twigs of (great) virtue (power, knowledge), usually of fruit-bearing trees, which were sacred to the Teutones. Such twigs were also known in Icelandic tradition. According to a brief passage featured in the *Lácnung*: "Were it Æsir shot, or Elves' shot, Or Hag's shot, now will I help thee," we see a descending hierarchy of spirit forms attributed to Scandinavian tradition. Disease erupts from the invisible wounds (bodily invasions) incurred from the mischievous and often malicious arrows that carried the flying venom of elves. Elf-shot[12] originates in Finnish tradition.

Native Teutonic magic and medicine can be distinguished from all other forms by its focus on the *wyrm*, specifically of venoms, elf-shot (flying venom) and to some degree, the doctrine of the nines, although, the latter two are not without external influences (primarily from Finland). *The Lay of the Nine Herbs* uniquely demonstrates how these elements coalesce. Woden too makes a rare appearance, confirming the provincial nature of this particular charm. As a narrative charm, it preserves a very specific formula, of expression, identification, and exorcism through repetition. Intent and outcome are clearly articulated.

Woden smote the serpent!

To accomplish this marvellous feat, Woden employs 'wonder twigs' (*wuldertánas*), that is, slips of wood imbued with the Germanic equivalent of 'mana' (*miht, mægen*). Being a virtue of his cræft and of the nine magical herbs cited in this charm, its efficacy in the repulsion and conquest of disease, is thrice amplified. Herbs believed to possess *miht*, were known as *lǽcewyrts*; a wyrt or wort simply means a plant used for food or medicine. King Alfred was a firm advocate of nature's ability to provide a range of medicines for human ailments and disease. Random words in Arabic (Celtic or even Hebrew) occasionally appear in some texts, especially in the *Lácnung* (and *Lorica*) which is an indication of the movement of copied documents across Christendom, and not necessarily always of peoples.

Anglo-Saxon literature was mostly written in the vernacular, as represented by the rugged lines of Beowulf and Cynewulf, the scholarly treatises of Aldhelm, history by the famous records of the Venerable Bede, and medicine by the Leech. Belonging to (the literary period commonly known as) the 'School of Alfred,' the widely acclaimed Leech Book of Bald, dating from around 900–950 C.E., is the oldest existing leech book written in the vernacular. Before its rediscovery, it was sheltered in that most romantic of all English monasteries, Glastonbury. Penned by a scribe named Cild, it is the oldest Saxon book dealing with the virtues of herbs we now possess. That the Leech Book was written in the vernacular is a remarkable achievement, indicating an assertive cultural trend to learn (but not to replicate) Latin scholarship, and to preserve that knowledge as supplementary to their own native knowledge. Dun and Oxa, are referred to as leech doctors who provided Bald with prescriptions. Probably written shortly after Alfred's death, this personal medical manual seems to be a copy of an older manuscript, written under the direction of Bald, who may have been a personal friend of King Alfred. Nonetheless, the position of the leech was subservient to that of the higher clergy, many of whom enjoyed a reputation for working 'miraculous' cures that corresponded to the Catholic liturgy, whereas, Leech Books by comparison, retain notable threads of Anglo-Saxon culture gleaned from the herb lore of our ancestors. There is certainly a wealth of native and non-native lore relating to plants, charms and charming traditions recorded there. Unsurprisingly, the longest chapter in the third book of the *Leech Book of Bald* is entirely dedicated to charms "against elf-disease."

During this early medieval period, the Church acquired and maintained a firm grip of its custodianship of the literary sources of medicine and magic, and as conversions became more commonplace, their knowledge merged with the common folk magics and healing or oral tradition amongst the diverse peoples inhabiting these Isles. The amount of available material from this period is lamentably small, and is often sketchy on medicinal advice. Medical knowledge was primarily the domain of monasterial clerics, as noted above, and while they treated the ravages of the world upon the human body, the human soul remained their principal concern. Afflictions were frequently perceived as just visitations for supposed sins. Advances in understanding the intricacies of disease and its causalities and cures was therefore excruciatingly slow and not without its theological resistance.

Moreover, owing to the influence of the English Church, allusions to the original Heathen spirits and presumed god-forms found within Old English charms are exceedingly rare. Ecclesiastical authorities austerely replaced every mention of former idols with various epithets for Christ (*Deus, Emanuel, or Adonai*) – who was believed to have especial potency to supress demons – his apostles, evangelists, saints (including Mary), the celebrated seven sleepers of Mount Celion and even certain Old Testament patriarchs and prophets. For this reason, a large number of the Anglo-Saxon spells contain invocations to all these forms, often indiscriminately. However, there are a handful of cases in which Heathen (elemental) spirits (including one to Woden) are propitiated.

Names carry magical significance. They represent power. It is apparent that peoples who demonstrate a propensity towards animism, prefer not to identify their higher spirits with direct names for fear of angering them; a name known, is a name used to gain power over that form.[13] For this reason, the use of mystifying names and epithets arose to protect both supplicant and spirit in all communications and exchanges. Whence those spiritual forms became deified, it was but a leap to apply taboos forbidding references to any 'deity' by name. Moreover, vernacular incantations, like Heathen rites, were summarily condemned; and, as in the case of the latter, substitutes were officially designated for the former. Sometimes the old charm rites were entirely dispensed with, and only the Latin prayer formulae remained.

Post conversion prohibitions placed upon the gathering of herbs, expressly forbade the performative action of galdor.[14] Former Heathen charming traditions for culling herbs were gradually replaced with Paternosters, Creeds, psalms, masses and other holy prayers in their stead, hence we find curious, incongruous liturgical formulas of all kinds (including Latin interpolations that were substitutes for forbidden names) within the Old English spells during the period of transition. Advocated as the only true cure, prayers replaced many Old English spells, charms and incantations in later general use. Of these, for example, the 'Prayer of St. John,' is declared as a cure for snake-bites. Such prayers were officially labelled *"Benedictio Herbarum,"* *"Benedictio Potus,"* or *"Benedictio Unguentum,"* according to their intended use in connection with herbs, medicines, or salves.

Teutonic folk-lore was subject to considerable revision and substitution throughout the medieval period. A 13th century German manuscript contains specific directions to priests for dealing with popular charming remedies and for altering spirit names found in Heathen invocations. By this time, the wind-elves were no longer implored for succour in a storm: petitions were addressed instead to the newly appointed 'water' saints (*wazzer heilige*). The pale semi-divine women whose appearance be-tokened good fortune to their beholders, were, in later legends, changed to nuns. In a Scandinavian song dating from the 10th century, Christ, like Þör, was acclaimed as the conqueror of mountain giants; his throne was placed at the sacred fount of the Norns. Possibly most striking of these changes was that of the genuflection, the Christian blessing made with the sign of the cross, where the sign of the hammer (which could have been runic in form) had been the old Heathen mark of consecration amongst Teutonic peoples. Signs and symbols were highly regarded in the Teutonic culture. Their applications are legendary, in the literal and figurative sense.

In *Sigrdrífumál*, 14–20, we learn of the origin of the runes, and of their usage and application as symbols inscribed, then 'scraped' off into water, mead or beer to be imbibed as a magical tonic or remedy. This procedure was adapted for use, enforced by words from within the Christian liturgy which replaced the Heathen incantations. A popular 'charm' used by Church clerics against demoniacal possession (*deófolseócnes*) by 'elves,' required up to fourteen unusual herbs that were steeped in hallowed water and placed beneath the altar for nine days, receiving nine masses. The infused liquid was used to make a holy drink or lustration to purge the demonic 'elf' from the body. In other charms, Soap, like wax and butter provided a medium for poultices and ointments. Stone amulets were 'charged' in similar fashion.

Several Anglo-Norman lapidaries affirm a rise in the use of precious and semi-precious stones in magic and medicine, very much popularised during the Middle Ages. This continuance of a Classical style of prophylactic and amuletic healing had more or less bypassed the Anglo Saxons, who'd inherited instead a love of herblore from the regions of their continental origins. One recipe of note, sent to King Alfred from Helias, the then Patriarch of Jerusalem, calls for a curious (friable) white stone. Observe how readily it preserves the component of 'scraping' symbols of power (such as runes, often cited in AS charms, and in the sagas as used by Norse peoples.)

> The white stone is powerful against the *stice*, and against flying venom, and against all unknown maladies: thou shalt shave it into water and drink a large quantity, and shave thereto a portion of the red earth, and the stones are all very good to drink of, against all unknown things. When the fire is struck out of the stone, it is good against lightnings and against thunders, and against delusion of every kind: and if a man has gone astray in his way, let him strike himself a spark before him, he will soon be in the right way.[15]

Similar charms to *The Lay of the Nine Herbs* use short twigs (*táns*) for transference of disease to running water. The *táns* are first scored with a name or word of power, smeared with the victim's blood, and thrown over their shoulder, or between the thighs into a stream of running water.

Certain herbs once regarded by the Anglo-Saxons with great veneration and reverence for their medicinal properties, are now almost forgotten. The common betony, for instance, once credited with extraordinary virtues, was recommended in no less than twenty-nine different diseases, yet is largely overlooked in modern herbalism. Vervain (Verbena officinalis) once regarded as a magical plant throughout the Middle Age, has also lost its former popularity. Despite this loss, it has been pointed out by eminent authorities that the Anglo-Saxons had names for, and used, a far larger number of plants than the continental nations, though (as noted) not all of them were understood. In their herb gardens, alongside rue, hyssop, fennel, mustard, elecampane, celandine, lupin, flax, rosemary, coriander, savin, and many other worts, whose virtues were proven, they also grew marigolds, sunflowers, peonies, violets and gilly-flowers, forming the origin of the English cottage garden. Their practical knowledge of gardening not-withstanding, the Anglo-Saxons had garnered their *materia medica* chiefly from the native herbs that grew around them, and their knowledge of herb-lore, or 'wort- cunning,' was evidently considerable. Herbs cultivated herbs for medicinal purposes were freshly gathered and also dried for later use. In this activity, we find the origin of the word *drug*, which was derived from the Anglo-Saxon word *'drigaji'* – to dry. As we have learned, they supplemented their knowledge of herblore with that of Classical botany which collectively formed the basis of English medicine from the Middle Ages, lasting to the end of the 17th century, at which point it was radically revised.

Nevertheless, it is worthy of note that many of the worts employed by the Anglo-Saxons a thousand years ago are still used in medical practice at the present day, especially amongst herbal practitioners. And it is in this field of operative herbalism, the author of this book excels, and will prove invaluable in theory and practice. Understanding the applications described here, of the nine herbs highlighted in this famous lay, will serve as an excellent primer for all other herbs found in popular use a thousand years ago. By providing this historical context for the remarkable explanations of the charms given by the author, a fuller understanding of their mechanics can be acquired. Culture and magic do not thrive in isolation, ignorance, nor neglect.

Shani Oates, Easter, 2024.

Endnotes

1. Elliott Van Kirk Dobbie, (Ed.) The Anglo-Saxon Minor Poems. Anglo-Saxon Poetic Records, vol. 6. (New York: Columbia University Press.1942)
2. It is especially a joy as I am currently researching this and other AS charms for my own forthcoming publication.
3. The texts of the early Anglo-Saxon practitioners were written in both Old English and Latin. The Old English medical manuscripts, for the most part, are merely translations of the Latin works.
4. Dysentery (the bloody Flux) and Typhus were especially rife. Several Anglo-Saxon words within the Leechbooks testify to a known range of maladies of this type.
5. J. H. G. Grattan and Charles Singer (Eds.) Anglo-Saxon Magic and Medicine; illustrated specially from the semi-pagan text Lacnunga. (Oxford: Oxford Uni Press. 1952) p107, note 4.
6. Grattan and Singer, 1952. pp152–3.
7. Wilfred Bonser. The Medical Background of Anglo-Saxon England: A Study in History, Psychology, and Folklore.' (London: The Wellcome Historical Medical Library, London, 1963) pp317–318.

8. Grimm, Jacob; Stallybrass, James Steven (trans.), Teutonic Mythology, G. Bell & Sons 1888 vol iii, p1211.
9. T. F. Thistleton Dyer, The Folklore of Plants (D. Appleton and Company, 1889.) p54.
10. Look to the *Canons of Edgar*, 18; *Theodore's Penitential*, I. i.4.; and Bede, *Eccles. Hist.* ii. 13.
11. Hence the later works of Snorri Sturluson gained significance as the preserver of such literary (skaldic) arts.
12. OED = shot is a sudden, sharp pain.
13. Claims to knowledge of supposed 'secret' names gave conjurers and magic workers a means of control and dominance for thaumaturgical operations.
14. The twenty-third Penitential of Archbishop Ecgbert.
15. *Leechbook II*, lxiv. (Bald)

Introduction

The Healing Charm
(Modern English Stylized Translation)

*Remember, Mugwart,
what you brought to pass,
what you readied,
at Regenmeld.*

*You're called Una, that most ancient plant.
You defeat three, you defeat thirty,
you defeat venom, you defeat air-illness;
you defeat the horror who stalks the land.*

*And you, Waybread, plant-mother!
You're open to the east, yet mighty within:
Carts creaked over you, women rode over you,
over you brides bellowed, over you bulls snorted!*

*You withstood it all—and you pushed back:
You withstood venom, you withstood air-illness,
you withstood the horror who travels over land.*

*Now, this plant is called Stune, she who grows on stone:
She defeats venom, she grinds away pain.*

*She's called Stithe, she who withstands venom;
she chases away malice, casts out pain.*

*This is the plant that fought against the wyrm.
She is mighty against venom; she is mighty against air-illness;
she is mighty against the horror who travels over land.*

You, Venom-loathe, go now!
The less from the great,
the great from the less,
until for both he receives a remedy.

Remember, Chamomile,
what you brought to pass,
what you accomplished,
at Alorford,
that no one should lose their life to disease,
since for him Chamomile was prepared.

Finally, this plant is known as Wergulu,
who a seal sent over sea-ridges,
to aid against venom.

These nine plants defeat nine venoms!

A wyrm came slithering, and yet he killed no one,
for wise Wōden took nine glory-twigs
and smote the serpent,
who flew into nine parts!
There, apple overcame venom:
There, the wyrm would never find shelter.

Fille and Fennel, a most mighty pair!
The wise lord shaped these plants,
while he, holy, hung in the heavens,
he sent them from the seven worlds, seven ages of man,
for wretched and wealthy alike.

She stands against pain, she stands against venom,
she is potent against three and against thirty,
against a foe's hand, against great guile,

against malice and bewitchment
from animal and spirit.

Now! May the nine plants do battle against nine glory-fleers,
against nine venoms and against nine air-diseases,
against the red venom, against the running venom,
against the white venom, against the blue venom,
against the yellow venom, against the green venom,
against the black venom, against the blue venom,
against the brown venom, against the purple venom,
against wyrm-blister, against water-blister,
against thorn-blister, against thistle-blister,
against ice-blister, against venom-blister.

If any venom comes flying from the east,
or any comes from the north,
or any from the west over folk!

Christ stood over illness of every kind.
Yet I alone know water running
where the nine serpents' guard.

Now, may all plants arise,
seas ebb, all salt water,
when I blow this venom from you.

Ingredients: Mugwart, Waybread open to the east, Lamb's Cress, Venom-Loathe, Chamomile, Nettle, Sour-Apple-of-the-Wood, Fille, and Fennel. Old soap.

Prepare and apply the salve: Work these plants to dust and mix them with apple mush. Make a paste of water and ashes. Take Fennel and mix the plant into the boiling paste. Bathe the wound with an egg mixture both before the patient applies the salve and after.

Sing the above galdor over each of the nine plants. Sing the galdor three times before the patient self-applies the salve and sing the galdor three times on the apple. Sing the galdor into the patient's mouth, sing the galdor into each of the patient's ears, and—before the patient applies the salve—sing the galdor into the patient's wound.

The *Nigon Wyrta Galdor*, (Nine herb charm, The Healing Charm) is a spell for healing a variety of complaints such as wounds, diseases, and poisons in humans and livestock. It was translated from the old manuscript Harley MS 585 (ff 160r−163r), Lacnunga (Old English 'remedies'), stored in the British Museum and is believed to date back to the 9th and 10th century. For this book, I have included the Modern English stylized version above. However, I have included the website for the translation of Old English: Normalized from Manuscript and the Modern English direct translation from Mimisbrunnr, *The Development for Ancient Germanic Studies* for anyone who wishes to study them in detail.

The text itself was part of a large body of work consisting of around two hundred remedies that included the use of herbs and spells. Unfortunately, the manuscript is difficult to translate. It is complex, is missing words, and other words may not have been translated correctly due to them falling out of use as the language evolved. Modern English has become a complex language over centuries. In modern terms, some words are specific in describing something, where its translation into the older tongue would have a range of meanings ascribed to it. Take the word Herb, it did not exist in the ninth and tenth centuries.

The translation during that period was conducted by Christian scholars who were faced with the difficulties described above, and also overlayed some of the original pagan content to fit in with the religious framework of the time. This is why Woden and Jesus cam be observed sharing the same Galdor.

While in this book Nine Herb Charm and Healing Charm are used as titles for the work, it is known by other names from different sources who have attempted to translate it. We should also bear in mind the charm when referring to an herb may have highlighted a group of plants belonging to the same species with comparable properties. What was available in one region in abundance, may be scarce or non-existent in others. It was possible that the ancestors may have adapted the charm based on what was available to them. While combing resources for the book, some authors had different ideas when it came to a particular plant, sometimes overlapping two or more species in their description and symbolism. This is especially the case with chervil. I have done my best to include these interpretations in the text.

The description and function of the herbs, if looked at closely, is anything but Christian. They were characterized as living beings with personality, experience, and supernatural abilities. These animistic qualities are present in everything in the natural world. The ancestors recognized this as a vital part of their own survival since primitive times. These beliefs were carried forward and made their way into the developing myths of the ancestral traditions.

For this book, I will be concentrating on the herbs we believe are described in the charm. While some of these plants are obvious, others are not. I will be looking at the physical characteristics of the herbs, origin and growth, and their symbolic, magical and culinary uses. This will enable the reader to build their own picture of the nine herbs and their correspondence to the nine worlds and its symbolism. While I have included correspondences recommended from various resources, I have included my own as well. Depending on the tradition and personal practice, my view of the observable universe is not identical to a person standing next to me and each reader will have their own view and insights so please bare this in mind. I have included tools in this work to assist the reader in enhancing their relationship with plants. While they may be useful to some, others may have their own practices. Keeping a journal on practices and experiences can play a vital role in this process.

Finally, the healing properties of these plants are a guideline. While they have been used for centuries and are currently being studied for their effectiveness in treatments, they should never be replaced by a professional medical diagnosis. They could cause allergic reactions and be incompatible with other medications and treatments a patient is undergoing. Not all herbs react well with others and may cause problems or cancel out the effects if more than one herb is used.

Gathering herbs must also be thought through properly. Unless someone knows exactly what they are looking for, it is advised to leave well alone. Some plants may be rare in some parts and illegal to pick. While anything by road and curb sides may be polluted and have unpleasant toxins, or animal, or human bodily fluids that would render them unsuitable.

Like humans, the origin of a plant will affect the nature, personality, and energies the plant possesses. A nettle grown in a city will feel quite different from one grown in a meadow. Spending time with the plant will help to get to know them on a deeper level. The best way to get to know a plant and it becoming an ally is to grow it from seed, nurture, and watch it grow.

The names Odin, Frigg, Freyr, and Frejya, among others who are considered the Gods and Goddesses in modern time are most likely natural spirits in ancient times whose identities and the correspondences we attribute to them today may have resembled something quite different back then, not to mention being known by a different name if they had one at all (e.g. Shani Oates in the foreword for this book.) We do not know for sure how old the Galdor is and whether it resembles what was translated in the tenth century. There may be a whole new language of symbolism locked deeper within the seed and roots of ancient memories that have been lost in time.

Why Nine?

If you knew the magnificence of the three, six and nine, you would have a key to the universe. – Nikola Tesla

The number nine was a sacred number to the northern peoples and even today is an important number in many magical traditions. Throughout the Eddas, sagas, and other myths, the number nine or multiples of nine is an obvious feature.

Nine is three times three, which makes it a triply powerful number in magical systems. Nine is associated with goddess energy. The Anglo-Saxons believed diseases were transmitted on the wind and that consuming these herbs would help guard and protect them from illness.

Woden took the nine glory twigs and threw them out into the world to give humans the gift of healing. There is even an instruction on how to prepare the plants into a salve. Woden/Odinn was instructed in the magical arts of Seiðr from the Goddess Freyja. The ancestors considered Seiðr to be an art performed by women only and not appropriate for men. In the Lokasenna, Odinn was mocked by Loki for this practice.

Odinn had an insatiable appetite for knowledge and wisdom. Through trial and experience he pushed the boundaries of forces and form to gain understanding and in a hope to overcome the ultimate ordeal, death. In his Mercurial form, he is an androgynous figure who has gone beyond human morality and the laws governed by the principles of matter, transforming into a superbeing. During Ragnarök, Odin was slain by Fenrir completing the final initiatory process that would have taken him from superbeing to become part of the universal consciousness. This is what the Volva from the Völuspá was trying to get across to him when he visited her. He was yet to understand the final initiatory step that had to be taken for that final transformation.

Nine is the last and highest single-digit number in the decimal system. In mathematics, nine is a composite lucky number and its divisors are one and three. It is a square of the third natural number and it is a third perfect square number in the number system. It is the first composite odd number which is the only single digit. It is a divine and the heavenly number present in the universe. The number nine is considered, enlightened transformation and an ending number. After nine, the numerical cycles begin again with new hope with the changes and modifications of previous errors. In numerology, the life cycles are measured in nine-year intervals. If you think back throughout your life there may be landmark events that would have coincided with these cycles and a pattern can be observed.

The number nine is unique. If you add the previous eight single digits together you would get 36, 3+6 is 9. You can add it, subtract it, multiply it, and divide it, the answer will always reduce to nine. Even zero has to obey the rule of nine. When we use multiplications of nine e.g. $1 \times 9 = 9$, $2 \times 9 = 18$, $3 \times 9 = 27$ and you have the patience to go on and on, you will notice the first of the double digits moving up and the second of the double digits reducing in sequence. This pattern is observed as the numbers triple and quadruple. A sequence of beginnings and endings.

Nine Herbs, Nine Worlds

These nine go against nine poisons.
A worm came crawling, he wounded nothing.
Then Woden took nine glory-twigs [wuldor tanas]
smote then the adder that it flew apart into nine (parts).
There apple and poison brought it about
that she never would dwell in the house.
Lay of the Nine Herbs and Lay of the Nine Twigs of Woden, University of Hawaii System.

It would be extremely easy to pigeonhole each herb in to one of the realms of the nine worlds. By doing this there is a danger of becoming too rigid in understanding the herbs themselves and their interconnected symbolism with one another. The nine worlds exist all at once. In the future, the now, the past, all at once and all the same. I invite the reader while reading this book to draw their own diagram of what they consider the nine worlds to look like and as they approach each herb, to immerse themselves in its symbolism in whatever practice they are most comfortable with and place on this diagram each herb and how they connect with the others. Like the Kabbalistic Tree of Life, a system will begin to emerge with connective branches into a living breathing organism.

Exploring the herbs and the nine worlds using this approach may bring a wealth of symbolism that is not apparent when viewing it from a practical perspective.

The Galdor

Using the Galdor, all or parts of it, may also add another dimension to the work. A Galdor should be sung, but I do not see any reason it cannot be softly intoned or recited like a poem if the original method is difficult or inconvenient.

We had the honour of being instructed in the practice of Galdor in its traditional form from Lars Magnar Enoksen for well over a year. It is not a straightforward process to begin with, but it is well worth the effort and an immensely powerful means of spell casting. The tone and pitch are as important as the words themselves. However, if this is not possible due to the proximity of others and not wanting to come across as a raving lunatic, then practice it in a low humming vibratory pitch. We lived in a property where, fortunately, our neighbours were at a reasonable distance from the house. However, we still made sure windows were closed when we practiced Galdor in its true form. We lived in a neighbourhood where people would not understand it even if we tried to explain it and did not want anyone calling the police because of a disturbance. However, one particular day I thought I distinctly heard someone go by and say "weird". If it is possible to go outdoors to a place where you will not be disturbed and weather permitting, then all the better. In fact, being in the open where there is nothing for miles and working with the force of the wind gives a more potent feel to the work.

If you place the fingertips on the throat, you are able to feel the different vibrations as each word unfolds. Pronounce each word slowly. When coming to the end of that word automatically move into the next and the next. At intervals inhale slowly allowing you lungs to prepare for the next part of the Galdor. With practice it is possible to be able to prolong the sounds of each word and make it your own.

Chapter 1

Mugwart (Mugwort)

OE Mucgwyrt (*Artemisia vulgaris*)

Remember, Mugwart,
what you brought to pass,
what you readied,
at Regenmeld.

Mugwart is a plant that grows in Europe, Asia, and the British Isles. Other names for this herb include felon herb, naughty man, chrysanthemum weed, old uncle henry, and wild wormwood. Since sailors smoked it instead of tobacco or cannabis, it was also known as sailor's tobacco. The edible parts are its leaves and roots.

Growing Mugwart

Artemisia, is believed to be native to most of Europe, Asia, and certain areas of Africa. These days it is found worldwide. It can be found in North America, but should not be confused with Western Mugwart, (Asteraceae), a member of the sunflower family, while the former is a member of the daisy family. Artemisia is a fast-spreading perennial, loving loamy, sandy soil. It is not a fan of poorly drained wet soils. Naturally it lives in forests, coastlines, fields and on roadsides.

Mugwart is distinctive from its stunning under leaves which are silver in colour with hairs that feel woolly to the touch. Watch them in a sunny day with a breeze, the colour shimmers and can be hypnotic. At the base of the stalk, the leaves do not have much depth, but the further up we go, the more numerous and directed they become evening out into a tapered point at the tip of the leaves. The leaf size can range from one to four inches in length, to three inches wide.

It flowers from late in July right through to September with tiny egg shaped yellow to reddish brown flowers in clusters that open from long threads attached to a hairy stem. Each flower is only about one eight of an inch big and are numerous.

They can be grown indoors and outdoors in pots, or grown directly in the garden. Pots are probably the easiest so the plants can be easily managed and do not grow out of control. They need cold temperatures to germinate the seeds. If grown in pots, or trays, sow the seeds on the surface of the soil, gently slide them in, but not too far and place them either in the fridge for a couple of weeks or put the pots near a north wall until spring arrives. Water the pots from the bottom to stop the seeds from washing away. To encourage germination, cover them with cling film or clear plastic ensuring they have plenty of light to grow. If sowing directly into the garden. Sow them in the same way as above water regularly until late spring when the plants can be handled transferring them to a permanent home.

Based on my own experience, using tap water for watering plants can be hit and miss depending on the level of mineral content in the water. Plants do prefer rain water, but if that is not an option, then fill watering cans and leave them for 24 hours. The chlorine in the water evaporates leaving it more suitable for plants.

Magical Use

Sacred to Woden, The Nine Herb Charm, The Healing Charm, calls it Una, believed to be one of the oldest herbs used by ancient peoples and considered it an extremely powerful one in magical practice and a powerful healer. In the verses below, we see the main power of this herb relates to strength, protection for travelers against a host of ills including wild animal bites and poisons, lightning, sunstroke, repels moths and other insects, even protecting against Troll shot, (A magical shot to cause harm from various spirits or forces in nature). It was taken as a tonic for those going on long journeys. Words were chanted while the tonic was taken.

Tallan te artemisiane lassus sim in via.

The herb was placed in the traveler's shoes prior to the journey. An old English Herbarium, presents another charm for protection of those carrying mugwart:

When someone wishes to begin a journey.
Have him this herb artemisia in his hand and have it with him.
Then he will not find the journey too great:
And it also drives off ill-will and wild trolls.
And in the house where he has it inside.
It forbids evil leechdoms.
And it averts the eye of baneful men.

Mugwart is one of the Artemisia family along with wormwood. I am mentioning these two because they are regularly confused with one another. They both contain thujone, an ingredient which is present in absinth, the drink which inspired nineteenth century artists, writers, and magicians. It is still unclear which psychedelic properties of absinth relate to thujone. We do know that the influence of absinth is generated after drinking it for nine consecutive evenings, if you can stomach the stuff that is. However, substances that contain thujone taken over an extended period of time and in large quantities may have toxic effects.

A spell to protect persons and the home from a terrible storm or extreme danger suggests throwing mugwart into the hearth fire or in a cauldron to keep everyone safe. For this reason, it was considered a women's herb. Used as an ally against dark forces by carrying some in a little pouch or concealed in an amulet. Placed at the threshold of the home, either hung in a bundle, or grown in a pot near the doorways. It can either be burnt as an incense, or mixed with water in a spray bottle, then sprayed, or smudged through the rooms of the house making sure doorways, windows, keyholes, plug holes, chimneys, and other points of entry as a method to clear the home of unwanted energies.

Burned as an incense, smoked, or drank in a tea with a little honey, it is believed to aid work in Seiðr, to enhance trance states, path working, clairvoyance, astral projection, psychic protection, scrying, and hag riding. It is even more effective if the work is done during the new moon and the Scorpio full moon.

This herb, like others in its category, can charge the physical space and is great for cleansing, clearing and consecrating temples, spaces, and any magical equipment. It is a suitable substitute for the sage smudge stick which is popular these days. Ruled under the signs of Scorpio, Capricorn, the planets Venus Neptune, and Saturn.

To help induce dreams, mugwart can be placed in a cushion made from two squares of black material stitched together. Leave one side as an opening and fill it with fresh herb, then sew it shut. Just remember it is there if you place the cushion inside your pillowcase. Cleaning the washer or dryer of mugwart because the stitching has come undone is not fun. These days capsules, teas and tinctures may be purchased to do the same thing when taken before bed.

It is believed to stimulate the *wod*, (inspiration), in the carnal arts when placed under the mattress or somewhere prominent in the room. Mugwart was also believed to be used as a component for lust spells. This may be due to its nervine properties that calms and relaxes the mind and body, removing barriers and inhibitions. In modern times, the essential oil is used to relax the brain, improving the circulation for the brain cells to receive much needed nutrients.

The name mugwart is derived from the old name mug weed which gives a clue to its use in ancient times. It added to beer and ale as a bittering agent before the use of hops.

Mugwart Smudge Stick

To make a smudge stick, gather three or four, six to eight-inch stems and place them together. From the bottom at the woody stem, twist the leaves around each other gently, but tightly. With red or white cotton, wrap the woody end thoroughly. continue to wrap the string with about an inch between each strand for the rest of the bundle, leave it to dry for about two weeks.

When ready to use, light the top letting it flame for about ten seconds. Blow out the flame and allow the smudge stick to smoulder. Have a small plate or traditional abalone shell for ash. It will continue to smoulder as you cleanse tapping the ash like a cigar. They are reusable, just make sure they are extinguished safely after use.

To Smudge or Not to Smudge

Everyone has their own methods and practices regarding ritual and ritual purification prior to a rite. Using a smudge to purify is a common practice during some group or solo workings. However, he planning a group working consideration should be given to those whose practices differ and have formulas of their own for ritual preparation. Their body of light may be properly prepared without being smoked. Just something to bear in mind.

Medical Uses

Mugwart resembles the chrysanthemum as well as ragweed. It's a perennial plant with green leaves that are narrow, deeply cut, and silvery on the underside, which gives its association with the moon and an herb used to aid the regulation of women's cycles, ease PMS symptoms, assist in hormone regulation, and easing cramps and pains when brewed in a tea and drunk three to four times a day.

It also resonates with Taurus and Libra relating to the midwives of old and new. Culpeper suggests a tea was believed to help aid childbirth and expel the afterbirth. This, however, may have only been used in the third stages of labour. In early labour it would cause considerable harm to the mother and child. Mugwart, as well as other plants like pennyroyal were used as an abortive, therefore it goes without saying that it should not be taken during pregnancy because it can cause contraction of the uterus causing miscarriage and avoid during breast feeding.

In Indo European tribes, a ritual was performed after the birth of a child by placing them on the earth. The midwife would walk three times around the child in a clockwise direction. This was done to assess whether the child was fit for life. Once this was done the child was lifted and presented to the sun or moon depending on when the child is born. The tribes believed that a child had three mothers. The birth mother, mother earth and the midwife who was in the centre of the other two, hence the name midwife. She was considered the connection to the ancestral spirits and were called upon on a regular basis being the holders of life and death in their very hands. The herb has a special connection to children and babies, it may be used in their blessing ceremonies. (*The Herbal Lore of Wise Women and Wortcunning*, Wolf D. Storl.)

In Europe and North America, it has been used to treat stomach conditions such as gas, colic, diarrhoea and constipation. It can also help with headaches, nosebleeds, insomnia, chills, fever, and nerve problems.

In traditional Asian medicine, it was used in moxibustion. Mugwart or wormwood leaves are formed into sticks or cones around the size and shape of a cigar and then burned on or over an acupuncture point to release energy. It claims to warm and strengthen the blood, while preserving the life energy. It is suggested that this method is used to treat cancers and inflammations. The smoke is said to improve the autonomic nervous system, having a relaxing effect on the body. It is suggested that mugwart contains antibacterial and antifungal properties. This claim has not been tested.

Chapter 2

Waybread (Plantain)

OE Wegbrāde (*Plantago major*)

And you, Waybread, plant-mother!
You're open to the east, yet mighty within:
Carts creaked over you, women rode over you,
over you brides bellowed, over you bulls snorted!

Plantain was called waybroad in ancient texts, because of its ability to grow in tightly packed soil by trails, roadsides, fields, and meadows. Originally native to north/central Asia and many places throughout Europe. The Latin name translates to sole of the foot due to it being found along the roadside. It was even worn on the inside of the shoe on the sole to prevent weariness while travelling. There are around two hundred species of the plant with just as many uses. The colonists brought plantain over to North America and it was introduced to the Native American people, who observed the way it grew and called it white man's foot. They, like the peoples of the plant's origin, realized the culinary and healing benefits plantain offered. The young leaves and seeds were included in their diet as well as used in pulses to help heal war wounds, soothe rheumatic pain, and draw out snake bites.

The English folk names associated with the herb are Cuckoo's bread, Englishman's foot, Leaf of Patrick, Patrick's Dock, St Patrick's leaf, Ripple Dock, Slan Lus, Snakeweed, and snake grass. The latter two names correspond with the plants flowers which when in bloom raise upwards on stalks resembling tiny serpents. It is not unusual for plants to be given a multitude of names. The names are sympathetic to either its appearance as our ancestors viewed the physical and spiritual world in symmetry, or the names were a clue to their beneficial or dangerous effects when brought into contact with humans and animals.

Magical Use

The Anglo Saxons called it waybread, Mother of herbs. It is feminine with the planetary association of Venus and element of earth. Waybread has the power to withstand and rush against its enemies. The mother has always been considered a symbol for protection and healing. Her womb protecting them until they are born and her role in raising them until they can do it for themselves. She will also fight to defend them no matter what the risks are to herself. It was gathered by people who wanted to conceive and birth a healthy child. Plantain's protective power may also be considered working in the realms of restraining and curbing, for the powers that can assist us have a broader and sometimes opposing effect depending on the way this power is viewed and the cultural laws of a place and tribe.

In sympathetic magic the herb was used for protection, strength and healing, especially as a snake repellent, by carrying in the pocket while travelling. Like mugwart it can be placed in a bag or made into an amulet and worn on the person or hanging in a vehicle to protect against evil spirits and ill fortune. It can be used in a potion for fever, tied with red cord and placed on the head to remove headaches.

Medical Use

All parts above ground are used in natural medicine. It can be made into pulses, tinctures, teas, salves, and washes. It is also interesting to note that plantain contains polysaccharides, when mixed with water it swells and has an emollient effect on the oesophagus and the stomach intestinal tract allowing evacuation. It can help sooth sore throats caused by repeated coughing. This is achieved by the mucilage smothering the bacteria. Natural Living Ideals has some suggestions for practical uses for plantain and gives instruction on how to prepare the plant beforehand. The right species of plantain needs to be selected, as well as the correct amount of water has to be observed to be used safely.

A poultice may be applied to ease burns, with a salve applied as aftercare. Fresh crushed leaves can be used to stop bleeding from fresh cuts. Wash with plantain tea or diluted tincture (1 tbsp to a glass of water) to prevent infections and promote healing.

Use 1 tbsp of tincture diluted with a cup of water for mouth ulcers and gargle. A tea may also be made for this and other ailments of the mouth and throat using 2–3 teaspoons of the dried herb in boiling water. Leave it to rest for ten minutes, then strain and cool. Take 5–10 drops of tincture under the tongue and ingest it slowly for sore throats and throat infections.

It may help to clear dandruff by applying plantain tea or oil infusion to the scalp and washing it off after an hour.

For poison Ivy/oak; Apply a poultice immediately, and then wash the area with plantain tea. Apply sludge afterwards until the stinging stops. Sunburn can be eased by applying a fresh poultice or plantain sludge liberally. Wash the area with the tea and then apply the salve.

It is a great tonic and cleanser for the body and useful for clearing the liver and kidneys, by drinking 1–2 cups of the tea daily, especially during the spring. For relief from gastrointestinal inflammation – Take the tincture under the tongue or drink in a tea. The essential oil may be useful in removing, or aiding the removal of splinters or broken glass that has been caught in the skin. It sooths dry sinuses, cold/flu respiratory infections and aids the digestive system. Take the tincture under the tongue or drank in a tea sweetened with honey.

Whether we consider a plant's use for food, in healing preparations, or magical work, it is important to remember

they have a living spirit, (plant wight). Plants and trees, like everything else in the natural world, have affiliations with deities and spirits. Our ancestors were aware of this. We do not have to look too far to see the many rites and customs honouring them alongside the seasons and the respective forces they represent. Many of these rites still exist around the globe. Some of which have been transformed over the years to fit into a modern framework of traditions and beliefs. While others have faded into superstition that individuals still perform whether knowingly, or on a subconscious level.

For example, gathering herbs on the eve of the summer solstice are considered to have properties considerably more potent than if they were gathered at any other time of the year. When Christianity became the dominant religion. St John became the patron of the date June 21st. The custom of gathering herbs on St John's even still continues up until this day regardless of whether individuals consider it a superstition, or believe in the powerful magical significance this time of year possesses.

Another summer solstice tradition in Europe was an ancient water rite which had its origin from pagan times where girls would make wreaths of nine herbs and flowers and attach a lit candle to them and cast them into the water to gain favour from the water spirits. This over time became a means for predicting marriage. If the wreath flowed downstream, the girl would be married that same year. If, however, the wreath would pin in circles for a while, she would be single for longer.

Some of these pagan rites were converted into practices against witchcraft and continued into the modern day to avert bad luck and bring in good fortune. A mugwart garland thrown on the midsummer bonfire would remove any ill fortune for the next year and protect the thrower from witches. Nowadays it is made into a smudge stick or just burnt to remove any unwanted energy and Betony had become very popular against witches and witchcraft, so much so it was planted on many church properties. Nowdays it can be planted at the threshold of homes keeping out unwanted people and forces.

It really is time to turn the tables on superstition and look at the value these herbs were to the ancestral peoples of the north.

Asking permission beforehand, whether performing an elaborate ritual a simple spell, or just asking permission directly can go a long way in providing a connection to the plant being worked with. We may also consider leaving an offering of plant food or water when we have completed harvesting, to encourage the growth of our own gardens or as an offering to the plant and land spirits for continued growth, protection, and prosperity. A gift calls for a gift.

Saying thank you before a meal, or a short verse of gratitude is a simple way to show appreciation to the spirit which embodies the plant. A spell can also be included to enhance the healing and magical properties of the plant in question. There are so many ways appreciation can be shown.

Chapter 3

Stune (Watercress)

OE Lamb's Cress (*Caradmine hirsute*)

Now, this plant is called Stune, she who grows on stone:
She defeats venom, she grinds away pain.

Watercress, also known as Lamb's cress, originated in Europe and southwestern Asia and was later naturalized in America. It is possible that it is one of the oldest sources of vegetable foods consumed by humans. The Romans were a big fan of watercress in their diet, while also using it in their own healing preparations. The Roman army was fed on watercress as a major source of nutrition, while working class folk would eat watercress sandwiches as a staple. For a short while it went out of favour but has again become popular in recent years for its nutritious benefits, becoming one of the new super foods.

This easy to grow perennial does not necessarily need soil and can survive in head waters, chalk streams, or brooks. It has hollow, sappy stems that float in the water with broad almost round leaves above the surface. In late spring/early summer, it will produce white flowers which attract a host of insects. Later, yellow seeds appear in long pods that resemble horns. It is cultivated in both gardens and mass produced for the general market.

A member of the Brassicaceae family, it is closely related to garden varieties such as radish, wasabi, garden cress, mustard cress, cabbage, cauliflower and sprouts among others. Watercress is 95% water with only small traces of carbohydrates, fat, protein, and dietary fibre. Rich in vitamins K, A, C, B6, calcium, magnesium, riboflavin and low in calories. The taste is a sharp mustard like flavour that is an excellent ingredient in soups, salads, sandwiches, stir fry and garnishes.

Magical Use

In the Galdor it was called Stuna, but it was also given the name Combat. This is due to the healing properties connected with this plant. When the poem talks about fighting with the serpent, this term refers to fighting disease, poison, and infection.

> "Combat" (Lambs Cress) this herb is called, it grew on a stone;
> Stands here against poison, stands here against pain
> "harsh" (Nettle) it is called, withstands against poison,
> Expels against wrath, casts out poison.
> These herbs have fought with the serpent;
> They have might against poison, might against infection,
> Might against the enemy who travels over the earthy.
> Heathen Anthology: Volume One. Valarie Wright.

Nettle and watercress embodied strength might and protection against the everyday ills the ancestors faced, the same remains true today. The rhyme also tells of ailments carried on the wind. They understood some diseases were air born and transmitted in this way from host to host.

Watercress is dominated by the moon, where the magical effect of any working is slow and subtle to begin with through a fluid energy which can transform one thing into another. The nature of the moon is tough, extremely cold, and dark. It is only the reflection from the sun that allows the moons rays to cover the earth. Water may move fluidly like a stream, travel lightly through the air as hot, moist, steam, but can also be solid and cold like ice.

When eaten it has a peppery element with a slight bite to it to give it its fiery elemental nature. This plant having a dual nature can correspond with more than one of the nine worlds.

We should not forget Ginnungagap, the primordial magical void from which creation was born into existence.

Exercise

There are various methods to enable one to connect with the spirit of a plant and using our own senses is the simplest. Taste, (gustation) and smell, (olfaction) are called chemical senses because both have sensory receptors that respond to the molecules in the food we eat or in the air we breathe. It is believed these senses are evolutionary, allowing humans to identify toxins and bad foods that can cause sickness and death.

People use all five senses when tasting food, but taste is the least studied out of all of them. Human taste can be reduced to the basic five taste qualities of sweet, sour, bitter, salty, and savory. However, there is more to taste then the five qualities listed. Studies by The Human Genome project and other biologists have identified the G protein receptors (GPCRs) which transmit information from the cells exterior environment to the interior providing it with information to perform its task. These cells are believed to make up the sweet, savory, and bitter receptors.

We are not clear in humans, if the transient receptor potential ion channels, which are evolutionary membrane channels, mediate the salty and sour qualities. There are Taste receptors located throughout the body and are believed to be involved in many of these processes. Researches are suggesting there may be interplay between chemical sensing in the periphery, between cortical processing and performance and physiology.

The exercise below is to focus the senses on taste. The experience may be more powerful without sight as a guide. There are restaurants that serve food in the dark to enhance the dining experience. Everyone's sensory experience is different, just as the results from the exercise. There are no right or wrong answers.

Find a time where you will not be disturbed and switch off any devices that may interfere with your work. Have with you a piece of watercress and a soft scarf. Sit comfortably and recite the verse from the charm:

> *Stune is named this wort, she on stone waxes; stands she against venom, stuneth, she against pain. "Stiff" she is named, withstandeth she venom, wreaked she the wrathful, warpath out venom.*

If you have a good memory, you can keep reciting the verse silently in your mind as you tie the scarf around your eyes and place the plant on your tongue. What are the sensations you get from gently rubbing the herb on the roof of the mouth with the tongue? How does this translate to the other senses and the rest of the body? What are the sensations when the herb is swallowed? Keep a record of your experiences in your journal.

Medical Use

Watercress is high in vitamin C and was a tonic for scurvy as an antiscorbutic. Another plant that was used for the same purpose was the European Plantain, (plantain major). Already we can begin to see connections between the herbs used in the charm.

Containing antioxidants, it can be added to pottage, (a thick soup), salads and stews to cleanse the blood in spring. Watercress contains nitrates like other green leafy vegetables and beetroots. It may aid the reduction of high blood pressure as part of a balanced diet and could be used to stimulate the appetite.

A poultice could be made to help rheumatism and skin disorders. The juice, if squeezed onto a wart, will aid in its removal. In many of the texts I have read, the properties in watercress and other varieties in the same family contain pain relieving effects. For coughs and bronchitis, the herb may be mixed with honey and used as a cough medicine. It may also aid in helping combat side effects in cancer treatment, however, more studies need to be complete before it can be said with any certainty.

Other sources suggest it aids the removal of gallstones and bring on menstruation. It may also help in the treatment of ulcers. The flowers and leaves are bruised, and applied to the skin helps in the removal of freckles, pimples and spots when used on the skin. Soaking and bathing in the leaves, flowers or a tincture may relieve a dull and drowsy disposition and lethargy. The juice helps to cure, acne, eczema, ringworm, rashes, and similar skin irritations and infections.

In the *Botanical Safety Handbook*, this herb, along with many others, are listed as not suitable as a treatment during pregnancy unless otherwise directed by an expert qualified in the use of the substance. It is unclear if the authors of some of the remedies are based on actual clinical records, or theoretical grounds.

Chapter 4

Stithe / Venom-loathe (Betony)

OE Attorlaðe (*Stachys officinalis*)

She's called Stithe, she who withstands venom;
she chases away malice, casts out pain.

Betony (Wood Betony) is among six species of a genus within three hundred species of wild plants. On researching betony and wood betony it has been exceedingly difficult to find any individual classification for either and nine times out of ten they are written about together. For this reason, I will do the same.

Betony is known under many names such as Louisewort, purple betony, bishop's wort, devil's plaything and sometimes wood betony. They belong to the family Lamiaceae, (family of flowering plants known as the mint, dead nettle or sage family). Wood betony is widespread in eastern North America, ranging from southern Canada (Quebec to Manitoba) south to northern Florida and west to eastern Texas. It can be found growing throughout northern and southern Europe and Asia,

Growing Betony

It grows in dry woodlands, sandy oak savannas, upland prairies, and in rocky riparian woodlands. Sometimes wood betony will persist in the lawns of infrequently mowed pioneer cemeteries. It can be found all over Europe in woodlands and meadows. Extremely hardy preferring heavy soil but wherever it grows it will grow profusely. Grows to a height of twenty-four inches and thickly spread to around ten inches. It is recognized by its dense spikes of pink or purple flowers, blooming from late spring to summer. The stems are aromatic, round lobed leaves with slight hairs. Some varieties of Stachys Officinalis in Europe have oblong, deeply edged, scallop shaped leaves of around seven centimetres long with bright magenta, rarely pink or white, flowers which protrude in oblong spikes in the summer. The chemical constituents of the plant are, Alkaloids (stachydrine and Betonicide), betaine, choline, and tannins.

It is easy to grow from seed. Sow in spring and summer covering very lightly with soil. It can be planted in trays, thinning and dividing when replanting in the spring and autumn. Divide the roots of the established plants, replanting at twelve inches from each other.

Due to growing so profusely, pots would be a better option with standard compost. However, they can make a spectacular feature near ponds and large borders. Cut back the flowering stems in the autumn and collect the seeds. Dividing established plants is best done during this time. It needs well drained soil and full or partial sunlight for the perfect growing conditions.

Magical Use

Betony/wood betony in the Galdor was known as the poison hater. Considered to be a cure against all poisons especially those of snakes and a cure for the bite of a mad dog. Betony was used as a protection from sorcery and witchcraft. Because the superstition surrounding the herb was so strong, it was used as a source for protection for centuries. Even Christians would plant betony within the church grounds and graveyards as a means of protection. By the tenth century it had become one of the most important magical plants. Several sources from old English remedies tell of how betony and rosemary were combined in an ointment for snake bites and was accompanied with this chant to remove general infection, puss, and other wounds represented by the serpent.

Early on Brigit's morn shall the serpent come from the hole.
I will not harm the serpent, and the serpent will not harm me.
Heathen Anthology: Volume One, Valarie Wright.

Considered an herb of Jupiter, the magical properties are used for purification, clarity and anti-intoxication. It also comes under the rulership of Mars for its ability to protect and defend. The protective element is especially useful to block outside influences, believed to protect the soul as well as the body. Carried on the person, it would help alleviate the darkest fears, especially those that are created by high emotional states, brought on by an overworked imagination. May be used in love magic, and spells to heal the body and spirit simultaneously. There is an old myth that if King Stag was wounded, betony is the herb that would heal him. It is a masculine herb, and the dominating elements are air and fire.

The Anglo Saxons used it as a cure for elf sickness due to its ability to block the influences and magic of hostile elves and other malevolent spirits. It was believed throwing betony at a Hedge Witch, would make her lose her way. It is used to block dreams or visions which cause disruption as well as preventing tormenting visions. It can be made in a tea to relieve spiritual and emotional confusion.

Placed around doors and windows it will protect the home from negative and harmful influences of spirits and other supernatural forces that may try to enter. Protection of the home can be re-enforced by growing betony in pots at the front and rear entrances and grown in the garden at the four quarters.

It can be boiled and used in the bath water to wash away bewitchment in children. At Midsummer it is traditional to throw it on the fire and then leaping through the smoke to cleanse and clear away evil and other ills.

Boiling and simmering herbs may be used as an alternative to incense, especially if anyone owns pets that developed anxiety due to the scent, and the smoke could be harmful for their lungs. Some rental properties may have a clause in their agreement against the burning of incenses or a home may have an oversensitive smoke alarm as I did in a former property. It was so sensitive, it went off every time I cooked anything.

Exercise

Take a large pan of water, bring it to the boil and lower to medium heat. Add three teaspoons of a single herb, any herb can be used provided it is not toxic, but the fresher the better. Alternatively, you can make a concoction of the nine herbs or any other blend you wish depending on your needs. The number three is sacred in many traditions. If you are combining the herbs from the charm, one spoonful of each will be enough. Stir it three times clockwise, three times anti clockwise and three times clockwise again (3 x 3 = 9). The steam given off will contain the scent of the herb and my husband and I have found it to be much fresher and more powerful for magical and spiritual work and uplifting the senses, than burning as an incense. Try and use freshly dried herbs if dried is all that is available, but they tend to lose their properties after six months. Keep an eye on the water ensuring it does not boil away and begin to burn the bottom of the pan. Using betony is an excellent way of clearing any malignant forces from the home.

Medical Use

Betony was believed to be a cure all, used in the treatment for migraine, indigestion and nervous complaints, staunching and healing wounds, sores, ulcers, and boils. It is a bitter, an astringent, a sedative herb that improves digestion and cerebral circulation. A nervine, excellent as a whole-body tonic. The Romans saw high value in betony, believing it to protect the liver. It may be employed as a tonic for a weak stomach, used when individuals find it difficult to digest meat, powdered and mixed with honey it can cure coughs, colds, wheezing and shortness of breath. A tea was made for chest problems and was considered useful against worms, jaundice, lung issues, fever, spleen problems, gout, dizziness, and epilepsy. Other conditions include, sinusitis, upper respiratory tract catarrh, gastritis, helps poor digestion, hypertension, and menopausal problems. can be used as a gargle for sore throats and gum inflammation.

As well as a cure for headaches especially those caused by nervous tension and stress, it may help improve memory, used for treatments for anxiety and neuralgia, by toning and strengthening the nervous system. A tea can be made by pouring hot water over one or two teaspoons of the dried herb.

You can make a simple medicine bag which can be carried around and placed under the pillow for stress relief, peace, and aid sleep. Inside a pouch place dried wood betony, lavender buds and rose petals. It is a simple bag to make, and all three ingredients are easily available. All three ingredients complement each other for the above afflictions.

All parts of the plant were used in treatments and its leaves and flower tips were used as a substitute for tea. Only the aerial parts of the herb are used these days and as a remedy it has fallen out of favour.

The external uses for betony may be used for wounds especially infected ones, ease insect bites, aids the healing of cuts, and ulcers.

The fresh plant produces a yellow dye which may be used as a hair rinse for greying hair. This is made from an infusion of the fresh leaves. The dried leaves like other herbs are used in herbal tobacco and snuff.

Chapter 5

Chamomile

OE Mægðe (*Anthemis nobilis*)

Remember, Chamomile,
what you brought to pass,
what you accomplished,
at Alorford,
that no one should lose their life to disease,
since for him Chamomile was prepared.

The Saxon word for Chamomile is Maythen and it is considered another heal all from the nine sacred herbs Woden gave to humankind. Chamomile was used in food and drink as a flavouring and a means to combat infections and other ills that our ancestors had to contend with.

Alorford the place referred to in the Galdor is now the village of Orford, off the Suffolk coast. It is a place that is known for its spectacular beauty with special conservation areas and is a site of scientific interest. It is split from the mainland by the river Alde and stetches to the Oxford coastline. connected to the coastal town of Aldeburgh. The southern Saxons landed in the area in the late 500s and could see the tactical advantage of the place. They named the area "the country of South folk". After the Norman conquest of 1066, Robert Malet a Norman nobleman and important landowner founded the town of Orford near a narrow stretch of land now called Orford Ness. This piece of land created a naturally sheltered harbor, and Orford flourished and became a very important trading post until the 20th century.

Remember, Chamomile,
what you brought to pass,
what you accomplished,
at Alorford,
that no one should lose their life to disease,
since for him Chamomile was prepared.
(Modern English Stylized Translation)

There are two varieties of Chamomile.

- German Chamomile, (Matricaria recutita), Ground Apple, Heermannchen, Camomyle.
- Roman Chamomile, (Chamaemelum nobile), Camomyle, Chamaimelon, Ground Apple, Heermannchen, (German), Manzenilla, (Spanish name), Maythen Whig Plant.

Their properties and uses are the same and their compounds are remarkably similar. There are one or two unique differences. I will include the names where these are necessary.

Growing Chamomile

Chamomile is an herbaceous plant that belongs to the Asteraceae family. Its origins are that of Europe, Asia, and North Africa, but now can be found throughout the world. There are several species of Chamomile, out of these we only use the two species I have given above. They differ in size, flower, leaves, type, and number of compounds that can be extracted for use.

German chamomile is an annual, (lasting only the year), while Roman chamomile is a perennial, (will grow back each year). The yellow centre of German chamomile is high domed, while the Roman variety has a domed centre that is lower and more rounded.

Roman chamomile grows up to twelve inches tall with fine, thread type green leaves and hairy stems. The flowers are a half to one inch wide with a fragrance like pineapple and apple. These days they are grown in Argentina, England, France, Belgium, and the United States.

German chamomile is taller, reaching 24 inches, having hairless stems with threadlike, sparse, and less ferny leaves than the Roman variety. The flowers are larger, and it does not spread quite as much as the former. The flowers are one to two inches wide and up to three feet tall having a similar smell to Roman chamomile when crushed. These days they are grown in Hungary, Egypt, France, and Eastern Europe. Their native distribution is Europe and northern Asia.

It is a venerable herb, well established as a plant healer, believed to bring health to a garden, with healing energies for all plant species, for this reason, chamomile is the patron herb for the garden. The white petals with yellow centres are a likeness to the sun. Our ancestors in modern Anglo-Saxon tradition referred to the plant as "Baldr's Brow" and were used in Summer Solstice rituals in his honour.

It is best when growing chamomile to start from small plants rather than from seed due to the difficulty in trying to germinate. If using seeds, it is best to sew them in a pot and cover lightly with soil during the spring or autumn months depending on the climate. Place them in a heated propagator until they are big enough to be transplanted into individual pots. The soil needs to be well drained and positioned where they can get plenty of sunlight. If they are solely for pots, then peat free compost is recommended. Once they become established, they are very hardy and require little maintenance. Chamomile is very difficult to grow in dry, hot climates. If the climate has cooler winters and very hot summers, it might be best to grow in a pot and kept in semi shade only exposing it to the morning sun while keeping it well watered.

It blooms in the summer and into the autumn in cooler climates and winter to spring in hotter ones. Roman chamomile spreads rapidly and is used as an attractive and more fragrant alternative to lawns. Before the Victorian era, when the lawn became popular, areas were covered with fragrant herbs that were hardy enough to trample on. A chamomile lawn is a suitable place to rest and sooth the body and mind. Lying upon it can bring on a relaxed and peaceful state. It may also be placed in between paving slabs and stones to add a more interesting look to any garden or yard.

Magical Use

The old year was divided into two seasons, winter and summer. Winter, beginning on the 1st November, and summer, beginning on 1st May. Depending on where in the region it was celebrated, the winter is of the Lady, (Freyja), ruled over by the Lord, (Frey). While the summer is of the Lord ruled over by the Lady. In the northern tradition, the days are marked by the solar Goddess Sunna and has masculine qualities, while the night sky is ruled over by the moon God Mani which is the feminine principle. This is the seed principle where everything is contained in the depths of its opposite. This is something to consider while dealing with old witchcraft laws, folk practices. Scott Cunningham describes chamomile as masculine with its element being water. However, it is strongly suggested that chamomile is feminine with its element being fire.

In later Anglo-Saxon times, people identified chamomile with Baldr, son of Óðinn and Frigg, a God of the Æsir who is the slain and resurrected God whose death is marked at the Summer Solstice. This is symbolic of the light season moving into the dark half of the year waiting to be resurrected at Yule.

Freyr, God of the Vanir, whose name means Lord, is God of sunlight who is reborn at Yule to carry the folk out of the dark half of the year and into the light of summer. His symbol is the phallus whose union with his twin sister Freyja brings fertility and life to the land enabling the crops to grow and animals as well as humans to thrive. He is the God of the harvest and the one to offer our thanks too at each meal.

In preparation for a ritual to Baldr or Freyr chamomile may be used in a cleansing bath for men prior to a ritual involving these divinities. It could also be powdered and placed on a charcoal disk and burned as an incense for cleansing or ritual purposes.

On the eve of the summer solstice men, women, and children in Poland would go to the field before sunset and gather chamomile, clove, and coltsfoot. These herbs were believed to have special magical properties when picked at this time to aid in the healing of rheumatism, arthritis, and lung problems.

Chamomile is known as the Goddess herb, connected to love, fertility, beauty, and sexuality. It was considered the mothers herb in witchcraft medicine, The name, 'Matricaria chamomilla', comes from Mater, matrix, mother. The ancestors used chamomile to stimulate the menstrual cycle and to help ease excessive menstrual bleeding while also relieving associated cramps. It was used to bathe women in the weeks following childbirth because of its antiseptic, anti-inflammatory, and soothing properties.

In early May, youths would collect colourful flowers such as mugwart, thyme, chamomile, sweet woodruff, ground ivy, bedstraw, and other aromatic herbs sacred to Freyja. They would build beds for love making in the meadows or moss groves.

Chamomile was one of the aromatic healing herbs added to the May bath where men and women would bath together to chase off the melancholy of the cold of winter. Love baths of the May season also contained chamomile as one of the sacred herbs used prior to their wedding to help the couple conceive a child. For modern ceremonies Chamomile may be used in the ceremonial bouquet, or wedding wreath as a symbol of love, union, success, and prosperity.

It is a symbol of success and material wealth. A few drops in a hand wash are believed to aid gamblers in luck before a game. It can be used in spells to enhance good fortune in all areas of life including legal matters. This plant is also a great herb to combat curses and spells cast against a person and property, giving protection, and purifying the space when sprinkled around the boundaries. Roman chamomile is especially useful as an ingredient in spells, oil, incenses, powders, baths and washes for longevity, love, and fertility, marriage, and sexual desire. Grow the plant in pots either at the entrance to the home, in conservatories on well-lit windowsills, or let it grow freely in lawns. There are many ways in which chamomile can brighten up the home and encourage, wealth, good health, and peace of mind.

Medical Use

Drink as a tea, followed by a relaxing, cleansing bath to help combat anxiety, clear and purify the body and the mind, and aid meditation. Added to a bath, handwash or even a general wash for the home to clean floors, surfaces and walls, it is easy to make. Boil the water and place in a bucket or bowl, steep for ten minutes and strain into another container. If the herb is unavailable, then a few drops of the essential oil may be used as an alternative. Using essential oils removes the need to strain anything and makes the job easier, A combination of herbs or oils may be used that complement one another providing additional qualities to the brew such as lavender, geranium, ylang ylang, among others.

As an essential oil, German chamomile is deep blue in colour, while Roman chamomile is a paler blue green that fades over time. Both are one of the few oils that are safe to use directly on the skin. I would still suggest a small skin test first for anyone who has not used it in case of any allergic reaction.

Chamomile tea is well known and used all over Europe for its treatment in digestive disorders especially German chamomile. It works best with its carminative, antispasmodic, antiseptic, anti-inflammatory, and mild bitter actions. Chamomile contains a presence of volatile oils containing many compounds including, azulene, which gives it its dark blue colour. Chamazulene is an aromatic compound which is a blue/violet and a derivative of azulene, which can be found in other plants. It also contains a range of sesquiterpenes, compounds known for their calming effects and supportive to the immune system as protection from harmful microbes acting as an antioxidant while assisting cellular repair. Other constituents in chamomile give the bitter principal flavones are glycosides that are used by many plants to store inactive chemicals. Chamomile contains salicylic acid which is found in many medicines to aid in the treatment of acne, by reducing swelling and redness. It is also used in the treatment of scaly thick overgrowths of skin such as psoriasis and other related skin conditions. Coumarin, is a type of anticoagulant sweet smelling with a bitter taste, These and other derivatives act together to create a well-rounded digestive remedy.

Chamomile has relaxing antispasmodic effects on smooth muscles and sooths cholic gently sedating the central nervous system and eases the impact of stress. It asserts anti-inflammatory effects on the gut providing anti-microbial action, (killing off microbial diseases), while increasing overall blood flow to the digestive system. These properties and more make chamomile a well-rounded holistic remedy for many conditions.

The Ancient Egyptians first recognized chamomile for its many healing properties, especially for its sedative, relaxing and soothing effects on the body and mind. In the 15th century, chamomile oil was being extracted in Poland for healing. Herbalist Stefan Falimierz, advised using chamomile to reduce eye strain and headaches, He believed if it was mixed with a small amount of wormwood, it would aid an easier delivery in childbirth.

The tea is a great drink to de-stress, relax and aid sleep. It is a nervine tonic and may be used to help relax the body dealing with conditions that bring on anxiety and panic attacks, shock, and confusion. There are studies that may suggest it can aid those with attention deficit disorder, (ADD), by counteracting the allergies that are associated with the disorder. Chamomile tea is recommended by herbalists for children who have difficulty sleeping. In a lab test, breathing in the vapours of essential oil reduces the production of adrenocorticotropic hormone, (ACTH), produced by biological stress and believed to help other forms of stress reducing drugs like diazepam making them more effective.

German chamomile may be used as a soothing bath to help calm and relax while helping sooth skin conditions. It may also inhibit the growth of underarm bacteria and may eliminate underarm perspiration. It is an active ingredient in some deodorants.

Used as a steam it can help with acne, colic, conjunctivitis, hives, and psoriasis. Chamazulene can prevent the formation of leukotrienes inhibiting the generation of toxic free radicals needed to trigger an allergic response.

It is believed to have regenerative properties. A drop on the skin maybe used to sooth small burns without scarring. Ointments and lotions containing chamomile are made to treat many skin conditions such as Eczema, chicken pocks, insect bites, dry irritable skin conditions, and a whole host of other skin complaints. Nappy rash creams also contain chamomile for its anti-bacterial and anti-inflammatory properties promoting tissue regeneration.

There are also creams with chamomile as an ingredient for cuts, scrapes, and abrasions by reducing the fluid from these wounds. A German study on patients who had undergone dermabrasion for the removal of tattoos had found creams containing chamomile helped reduce the amount of fluid lost and reduced wound size.

For twenty years the herb has been known to treat peptic ulcers. The anti-inflammatory and antihistamine soothe digestive tracts while helicobacter pylori one of the most common causes of peptic ulcers is counteracted. If there is concentrated pain from an ulcer than Chamomile tea with a high fibre diet can help alleviate the symptoms.

It contains apigenin chemical that prevents the production of proteins that allow cancer cells from anchoring to new sites. Apigenin can also counteract inflammatory reactions necessary for tumours to gain their own blood supply. It may also help with the condition lupus, the apigenin stops the formation of the tissue destructive hormone interleukin-8(IL-8). For irritable bowel syndrome, (IBS), Naturopathic physicians recommend the teas as part of a program.

Cosmetic Use

It is a key ingredient in some beauty products and cosmetics. It may help smooth the under-eye area while reducing dark circles. Body butters, body scrubs, deodorant wipes, shave gels, cleansing gels and facial wipes are found to contain chamomile again for its soothing and regenerative properties.

The Botanical Safety Handbook suggests chamomile should not be used during pregnancy unless otherwise directed by an expert qualified in the appropriate use of this substance.

Chapter 6

Wergulu (Nettle)

OE Aergulu (*Urtica spp*)

Finally, this plant is known as Wergulu,
who a seal sent over sea-ridges,
to aid against venom.

Stinging nettle, or common nettle, is native to Europe, Asia, North America, and North Africa. It grows and thrives in damp conditions, preferring a temperate climate. There are several other species worldwide that are related but are more of an exotic variation. Other species such as hops, and hemp are now considered to be separate species during recent classification. Their name, for the common stinging nettle species in the UK from the genus Uricia, the Latin name uro, to burn, speaks for itself. In old English it was called netele. Dioica means dioecious. The Greeks called it acalyphe.

Growing Nettle

It can grow up to seven feet tall in the summer but dies back in the winter. The rhizomes are bright yellow like the roots. Its leaves are green and soft ranging in size from one to six inches with serrated edges that gather into a sharp point. The flowers are a green/brown colour, flowering between July and October.

The hairs on the stems and leaves are both non-stinging and stinging, (trichome). These fine stinging needles break off and transfer to the individual person or animal being stung when they come into contact. The chemicals in the sting include acetylcholine, (a compound that occurs throughout the nervous system and functions as a neurotransmitter), histamine 5-HT, (serotonin), moroidin, (an active compound found in stinging plants), leukotrienes, (inflammatory mediators), and formic acid.

Magical Use

Some of these chemical compounds can be found in ant and bee stings. This gives them a connection to the Goddess Frigga. Bees are an emblem of women, the feminine powers in all its symbolism. Besides the obvious reasons why the bee has immense value to the survival of ourselves and other living creatures on this planet, if we follow these branches of thought in a meditation and what will be revealed is a much deeper universal connection to everything from that which is material and everything beyond it.

The northern European peoples considered this herb to be both a protector and able defender. This was most likely to be an accidental discovery when one of them had an encounter the plant and felt the results. Because of this strong connection with defence and protection nettle was identified with Þórr, (Thor) and was hung in the home to keep lightning at bay.

It may be used in knot spells to reverse curses and jinxes, sending the negative forces back on the sender. Used as an ingredient for incense, or to dress candles can promote personal power and purification.

Nettle as a protector and defender was combined in an herbal mixture to consecrate a ceremonial blade. The blade would be plunged into the mixture while hot rendering it blessed and consecrated by the Gods.

Carried in a bag, or sewn into a pouch and worn on the person, it was believed to protect against any curses that are targeted at the wearer. In some regional folklore it was believed it could dispel darkness. Combined in a tea with yarrow to strengthen the spirit especially when the individual had a fear of otherworldly travel. When it was spun into a garment, it was believed to protect the wearer.

For household protection, it can be sprinkled around the house taking care to include windows, keyholes and any area where there is a link to the outside. It does grow rapidly and may be grown in pots at the entrances of homes or boundaries inn gardens, so it does not grow out of control. Warriors would hang them in pouches before battle as a means of protection, but it would also ward off fear and negativity bringing a sense of peace.

Before cotton was introduced for household linen and clothing, nettle fibres were spun to create a fine fabric. The earliest evidence of nettle being used for fabric was from the bronze age era in Voldtofte in Denmark, (Barber), with further evidence found in cloth production from Scandinavia, Poland, Germany and Russia. Nettle, (nĕt'l), and needle, (nēd'l), were believed to originate from the Indo-European word, to sew. It was used as a green dye for clothing and for silk it produced a pale-yellow colour. Right up to and during the first world war it was used to dye military uniforms.

There is a fairytale written by Hans Christian Anderson called *The Wild Swans*, (it has other names and versions depending on the tale's source), involving nettle being spun into fabric for a magical purpose. Elisa, the only daughter of twelve children by a widowed king, was driven into exile when her new stepmother transformed all her brothers into swans. Fortunately, her brothers took her to a far-off land where she would be safe. She contacted the queen of the fairies who told her she was to collect nettles from a graveyard and spin them into shirts, while doing this, she is not to utter a word during the whole process. The conclusion to the story is she managed to spin the cloth into ten of the shirts but one of them was missing a sleeve because she nearly ran out of time before her brothers remained swans forever. When she threw the shirts on the backs of her brothers all were transformed back into men apart from one who had a wing of a swan. It is a story about self-sacrifice and how far a person would go to save the people they love despite any pain they may endure. An old English tale suggests that being turned into a swan is to lose your connection with the present and become disconnected from the earth. Being stung by a nettle really does bring us back to our senses.

While the act of weaving is believed to have been employed for textiles around 12000 years ago as a craft, humans have been weaving plant fibers such as twigs and branches to build homes and other useful objects for a considerable time.

Spinning is when natural fiber is spun into yarn and used for weaving and other useful tools. The origin of spinning is unknown, but there is archeological evidence that may point to its early use around 41000–52000 years ago by Neanderthals using tufts of animal hair and plant fibers rolled together by hand along the thigh to create a type of chord.

What inspired humans to spin and weave may have come about through observations in nature, such as insects spinning webs and cocoons, or birds making their nests, or maybe it evolved through trial and error. Whatever the origin of this discovery had been, it became an important stage in human development and a skill we would be lost without today.

These myths and folk tales that have come to us have most likely been transformed over time and may not have looked like the stories we read today. These tales have a clear meaning behind them, but there may be some threads of ancient wisdom that is lost as these tales have evolved. Whether we are talking about the spider spinning her web, or the distaff, spindle, and spinning wheel, they always had a female as a central character. This was a woman's art that was and still is passed down from generation to generation. With it, other disciplines and traditions were passed down through word of mouth.

Myths tell of enchantresses and women alike using weaving to their advantage. It also shows a strong work ethic and an attention to the smallest detail. This type of sympathetic magic has been used throughout the ages and is another technique to harness these powers to great effect. It does not matter if the craft is sewing, knitting, embroidery, anything in this discipline. The repetitive actions can be either accompanied by a rhyme to which a goal is stated spoken aloud or silently. A rocking motion while doing this may also be included. When the process is completed there will also be something that has been beautifully created and a truly magical gift for someone. For those who are not creative in these arts, the plaiting of the hair may be employed for the same purpose, or the chord bracelets of assorted colours that can be found in many retail outlets. These kits come with many colours and selecting one that complements the magic being performed can add an extra dimension to the work being performed.

The Scandinavian Goddess, Frigg, has a close relationship with spinning. The constellation of Orion's belt was identified with Frigg's distaff. She spun the clouds in the sky and the perfect patron for her would be the sheep whose wool is spun into garments and household items. She is also aware of the fate of all things and therefore very familiar with the intricate formation and paths of the web of wyrd.

The Valkyries in Njal's Saga were described as women weaving on a loom, with weights of severed heads, shuttles made from arrows, and the human guts for a warp, of yarns or other things stretched in place on a loom before the weft is introduced during the weaving process). They would sing an exalted song of carnage. During the Pre-Roman Iron age, it was common for ritual spindles and loom parts to be deposited in a Dejbjerg wagon. Such wagons have been found in peat bogs in Dejbjerg in Jutland and believed to be associated with the wagon goddess.

Throughout many countries in Northern Europe, there are older Goddesses connected with the spinning wheel and the plough. They go by many names, among them are Frau Holle, Holda, Percht, Bercht, Herke, Harke, Herra and Werra. While the further North we encounter similar deities with names such as Frau Frekka, Frick, Frau Wode, Gode. All of these are named as the wives of Woden and accompanied him on the wild hunt. They would all visit homes during the twelve nights of Yule. She is looking for domestic order and whether all the spinning had been completed. She would reward those that had accomplished their work and would punish those that had not. If anyone wondered why socks were a popular Yule gift this could be the reason behind the tradition. Apart from being given something to help them through the cold winter, the idea was to use up all the yarn and thread before the beginning of the twelve days in order not to anger the Goddess.

The Norns, Urd, (what has been), Verdandi, (what is) and Skuld, (what is to come), are the three beings who crafts the fate of every living being including the Gods and Goddesses themselves. Noone escapes the fate which has been dealt. The spinning, weaving, and twisting of these threads are fed into the web of Wyrd and binds with the threads of all others that have gone before and those that will follow. All connected in a cosmic space where there is no space time and everything existing at once. This may be accessed through meditation, trance, or other means of bridging the gap between us and those beyond.

As a Shamanic tool, it may transmute painful life experiences into personal change and growth and help those who are dominated by their emotions and break cycles of unhealthy habits. As well as having a connection with the fire element, it is also governed by earth as a symbol of the Goddesses of nature and those of the underworld.

I grew up in what was at the time a small town in the United Kingdom. Back then, we had the pleasure of growing up among fields and brooks, where we would play for hours. When any of us got stung, we would find a dock leaf, (Rumex obtusifolius), growing nearby. We would either squeeze the juice onto the sting or rub the effected spot with the leave to soothe those little white blisters that appeared from the sting. It always worked for us and there is an old saying that where there is a plant that may cause harm, there is always a cure growing nearby. So far, there is not any medical evidence to suggest that this is an efficient cure for nettle stings. The dock leaves do contain an alcoholic alkaline which may neutralize the sting. I know it works and so do many people who have tried this method.

In folklore a bad spell could be broken by thrashing the individual that was under the influence of the curse with a nettle. There was a belief that rheumatism was a curse and so the area would be thrashed to remove it. In Germany this was called. Hexenschuss, (witches shot).

Medical Use

The Romans who were stationed in England and northern Europe would thrash themselves with nettle to improve the circulation. While in similar cold climates, it is believed to help relieve the symptoms of frost bite.

The formic acid from the sting enters through the skin to relieve the pain of the condition. In modern times there has been studies in the United Kingdom of treatment for osteoarthritis using nettles taken as an internal remedy and the fresh young leaves rubbed on the affected area. Many patients who were in the trial felt a significant improvement in pain levels.

When it is used in a soup, it gives it a fish flavour. This is probably why Alberrtus Magnus believed that mixing the juice of the nettle and that of the house leek and then placed in the water it would attract fish. It is known in a few sources to be an emblem of the fishermen in times of old.

A folk belief that a bowl of nettles placed in a room, or under the bed of a sick person, drives away influences that could have caused the disease. It is also suggested that picking a nettle by the root reciting the name of a person with a fever and those of their parents is a cure for their condition.

Pre-Christians and Christians both considered the nettle a symbol of the coming of spring. In Russia on Maundy, (Thursday), the people would use the green dye to decorate their eggs to celebrate the return of spring, Nettle was a valuable herb used as a spring tonic and could be consumed to remove toxins and clear the system of winter fatigue. It was the promise of spring and a symbol of joy. During the rise of Christianity, the old festivals where secularized and were incorporated into the Christian calendar where the custom of painting eggs became a symbol of Easter and man.

Picked with gloves and washed it is then boiled like spinach to remove the stinging hairs. It is rich in minerals containing calcium, magnesium, phosphorus, manganese, silicon, iodine, sodium, Sulphur iron, and a high content of vitamin C.

The young green leaves are great in salads in the spring. They were given to people in times of old as a recovery food for those who were chronically sick and those who were in recovery due to its rich vitamin and mineral content. The leaves were freshly squeezed and given to those who had an iron deficiency. They are best picked during June to October but recommend the young spring leaves for its nutrients. They are also excellent in stir-fry, soups and sandwiches. It can act as a general immune support.

There are recipes where nettle is used to make a beer. Eoghan Odinsson gives a simple recipe in his book, Northern Plant Lore.

Quantities of the young, fresh tops are boiled in a gallon of water with the juice of two lemons, a teaspoon full of fresh ginger and a pound of brown sugar. Fresh yeast is floated on toast in the liquor, when cold to ferment it. When it is bottled, it is a wholesome sort of ginger beer.

It was, and still is used to treat conditions such as anaemia, eczema, arthritis, gout, allergies, aid for general pain, cough, tuberculosis, an expectorant, and urinary tract disorder, among many other conditions. It is one of the most widely applied herbs in natural medicine. In modern times freeze dried or fresh extract may help conditions of the flu, asthma, mucus conditions of the lung, bronchitis, chronic coughs, colds, and pneumonia.

For the last few years, it has become a popular remedy for hay fever containing a natural antihistamine. For seasonal allergies start drinking cups of the tea two weeks before the spring buds come through. Tests and trials using the freeze-dried herb against the organic fresh herb suggest some of the properties have been denatured in the freeze-drying process. However, 58% of those involved in hay fever trials say the freeze-dried herb helped to alleviate the condition.

The seeds can help restore compromised kidneys. In traditional Chinese medicine the seed extract is used to regenerate the kidneys. It may also protect against drug toxicity, chemotherapy, and diabetes. Moroidin the compound found in the sting is being considered for a chemotherapy drug used to be an antioxidant against cisplatin an agent found in chemotherapy.

Donald R. Yance suggests that nettle leaf extract was studied for its effects on adenosine deaminase, (ADA), activity in prostate tissue taken from patients with prostate cancer. ADA binds and stimulates plasminogen, (the inactive precursor of the enzyme plasmin present in blood that leads to tumour growth). Extract from nettle induced significant restriction of the ADA of prostate tissue, which may be useful in suppressing prostate cancer.

It is good for hyperthyroidism and adrenal fatigue. It is a trophorestorative, (nutritive restorative for the body, usually to an organ to correct deficiency, not simply through stimulation but vital nourishment for the organ).

The tea may be used as a diuretic and energizing tonic. It can lower uric acid levels aiding the treatment of gout. Relieving the symptoms of eczema, it can have a firming and toning effect on the skin. It increases the flow of urine. It can also lower blood pressure, lower cholesterol, lower the risk of diabetes and has a strong association with combating heart disease. because nettle contains antihypertensive, antihyperlipidemic, (treat high levels of fat), and antidiabetic properties. There are some studies that suggest that the leaf extract may be useful for improving the symptoms of type 2 diabetes.

The compounds in the roots are believed to help alleviate symptoms of Benign prostate hyperplasia, this is a common condition as men get older. It is an enlargement of the prostate gland and can make passing urine uncomfortable causing urine to be blocked from flowing through the bladder. If not corrected this problem, can cause urinary tract or kidney problems. Nettle can alleviate the symptoms of this condition, but it is always a good idea to be checked out by a specialist to ensure there are no other issues that are causing the problem.

Used on the hair it may help to relieve symptoms of dandruff and oily hair. It can enhance hair condition for a healthier look. It is also help improve the condition of nails when taken as a supplement.

Chapter 7

Apple (Crab Apple)

OE Æppel (*Malus sylvestris*)

A wyrm came slithering, and yet he killed no one,
for wise Wōden took nine glory-twigs
and smote the serpent,
who flew into nine parts!
There, apple overcame venom:
There, the wyrm would never find shelter.

Crab apple or scrub apple, wood sour apple, malus baccata. are smaller parents of the larger varieties of apple that are available to us today and believed to be bred from these species for a hardier plant which is pest free and more commercially productive. In this chapter, I will discuss the apple in general and only refer to the crab apple where it is necessary.

There are many varieties of apples available today and there are several varieties of crab apple whose fruit range from sour and not fit for human consumption, to sweet varieties that are edible and useful in preserves, ciders, and stews. All apples belong to the Rosaceae, (rose family). This is an interesting point to consider with both having similar and, in some cases, identical symbology. Both have a unique beauty while having thorny stalks and ranches that can draw blood if not paying attention. They are considered to originate from the mountains of Kazakhstan, but it is unclear how and when they spread throughout Europe and Asia. Malus sieversii may be the key ancestor and could have been domesticated around 3000 to 4000 years ago. Three species may be considered native to the United States. Malus coronaria, M. Fusca, and M. ioensis, while others were believed to be brought to the United States by colonists through seeds and cuttings.

Growing Crab Apple

The European crab apple, (Malus sylvestris), the name meaning "forest tree" are found all over Europe except Iceland. It is a small, thorny wild tree which grows at the edge of forests, thickets, roadsides, and hedgerows. They can either be found standing alone, or growing together in small groups. It was largely planted in hedgerows during the enclosure years in England between 1604 and 1914. It is considered to be the contender for the domesticated apple, believed to have evolved around 1500 years ago This variety is considered the key ancestor for the crab apple rather than Malus sieversii. The tree can live from eighty up to one hundred years. It has a wide canopy with a height of ten to fourteen meters. The bark is grey/brown, and the wood is real hard wood. The tree, being exposed to the elements, can look rugged and knotty and have some irregular shapes. The twigs develop spines where the name crab apple may have been derived. It is a host tree to the mistletoe, (Viscum Album), and can be seen covered in lichens. The crab apple being a Goddess tree has a natural relationship with mistletoe. The latter is sacred to Queen Hel and in Traditional Witchcraft it is sacred to the Horned God as Holly King. In the spring they have brown pointed leaf buds which develop into glossy green leaves that are oval with rounded teeth about six centimetres long. The white/pink, sweet-smelling blossom appear in early to mid-spring, depending on the weather conditions. It is a favourite early flowering plant for bees when there is limited pollen around. The flowers eventually develop into yellow/green apples around two to three centimetres across. When ripe, the fruits may have flushed red or white spots. Besides pollination, birds and mammals eat the fruits scattering the seeds. This is a wonderful tree for our eco system, even planted in gardens it does not take up much room. Like any other fruit trees, they do need care. The woodier the tree becomes the less fruit it will produce.

This species has become rare even though it is widely distributed through Europe. It has become a priority species in the Nordic Wild crop conservation program. In Finland where it only grows in the southwest of the country, it has become a protected species. In Norway and Sweden, it may be found in the south of the country, while in Denmark they can be found everywhere. In the United Kingdom, they are distributed throughout the country except the far north of Scotland where the climate is not suitable. The biggest threat these native species face is hybridization. Many trees found in the wild have grown from self-seeded and reverted to a wild form of crab apple, or crossed with true crab apple varieties. The best way to be able to distinguish the true crab apple from other varieties is the closer to the parent apple, the larger and sweeter the fruit will be. Native sweet crab apple trees, (M. coronaria), grow in the mountains of North Carolina above elevations of around 3500 feet. They have beautiful orange/red autumn foliage on twenty to thirty feet tall trees with an extravagant spring floral display in mid-May. The rose/pink buds unfold to reveal an impressive display of delicate white flowers. This is then followed by yellowish/green fruit, "Charlotte's". The large crab apples eventually follow in late summer early autumn. This variety is great for making cider or preserves.

Transcendent crab apples, (Malus baccate), are a variety of Siberian apples. The pink and white blossoms have a sensational aroma, followed by a large 2-inch fruit with red-blushed, yellow skin. Their fruits are used in stews, ciders and preserved in the autumn.

Centennials, (Malus Domestica), are a very sweet, small, oval shaped fruit with rosy skin which ripen in August. In the spring the white blossoms bloom with an explosion of scent from pink buds. These trees have a thick green foliage and are great pollinators. It is an excellent fruit for preserves and a great fruit to eat raw. I could list other varieties but encourage the reader to explore for themselves.

Apple-crab apple crosses result in sweeter fruit and hardier trees than straight crab apple hybrids. These trees are also able to grow in zones where their parent varieties were unable to germinate. These varieties can be found at any good garden centre.

Crab apples, apples, and other related plants such as pears and cherries contain seeds with the compound amygdalin, a cyanogenic glycoside composed of cyanide and sugar. When metabolized in the digestive system, it degenerates into a highly poisonous hydrogen cyanide. However, there are factors that would make this unlikely. The amygdalin in the seeds is release when they are crushed or chewed. The human body produces HCN in exceedingly lesser amounts. A couple of seeds chewed will not harm anyone. Depending on the variety of the apple an adult would have to consume maybe 150 to several thousand seeds to be at risk of cyanide poisoning. The core and seeds of one or two apples will not cause any problems.

The apple is a symbol of love, youth, vitality, fertility, and sexuality. It also represents illusion, death, the realms of the underworld, initiation and regeneration. It relates to Goddesses in many traditions captured in the myths which have made their way into old tales and fairy stories up until the present day. The tree itself is considered a Goddess tree and was one of the seven chieftain trees under Brehon law. Like other sacred trees in Celtic law, unlawfully cutting the tree had a life sentence attached to it.

While at first glance the apple is related strongly with the water element with its obvious affiliation with love, sexuality, fertility and the like, earth features strongly with growth, vitality, healing, and its underworld persona of decay and regeneration.

Fire and air may also be attributed here, like all living entities we need the sun to survive and oxygen to breath which is produced through photosynthesis. Oxygen is a by-product of sugars and other compounds created when carbon dioxide and water are pulled through the leaves using the energy of the sun to convert them into useful products produced by the tree in a constant cycle. When cutting into the apple, the core resembles the pentagram which represent the four elements plus spirit.

Magical Use

The Norse Iðunn/Iduna goddess of immortality was the keeper of the apple. There is not much written about Iðunn, but her role was essential to the gods, being a protector of the apples of immortality that kept them youthful until Ragnarök. Without these apples they would age, become ill and eventually die.

In Snorri's *Ragnarok,* Iðunn, whose name may mean "again granter", was abducted along with her golden apples by Loki and the giant Þjazi. Without the apples the Gods and Goddesses began to age. They forced Loki to bring Iðunn and the apples back with the help of Freyja's falcon cloak, (fjaðrhamr), During the escape, Loki transforms Iðunn into a nut and carried her away while Þjazi was out in his boat. When Þjazi came home and found Iðunn and the apples missing, he noticed a falcon with a nut in its claws flying away. Þjazi, in hot pursuit went after them in the form of an eagle. The Æsir were finally able to kill the giant before he could reach Ásgarðr.

The story of Iðunn and her apples being abducted and spirited away to Þjazi's home in Jötunheimr, the realm of death, is just one of the Scandinavian myths dealing with the cycle of death and a journey through the underworld only to re-emerge through trials after a state of transformation. Even the Gods are not immortal and will face their fate at Ragnarök. However, from the aftermath a new cycle begins from the remnants of the old and will eventually be broken down and the whole process starts again. This story is echoed on a cosmic level with stars, planets, and anything else out there coming to the end of their life and being transformed into something else in a chemical process that takes millions of years. On our planet we see this process in everything right down to the smallest grain of sand.

The frost giants desire the gifts of the gods and will use any means to acquire what they want. Loki, who initially was a God of mischief, later becoming something more sinister, was the culprit behind most of the trouble and is forced by the Gods to amend the situation, usually under the threat of pain or death by Þórr. This and other myths like them show the symbiotic relationship as neither can exist without the other. The eagle, (death), will always chase life but life must surrender to death and defeat it to transform and evolve.

In the practice of Seiðr, the concern is not with the death of the physical body, but a spiritual death that leads the soul to enlightenment through a variety of initiatory processes. The Völva and Vitki perform rites and rituals taking an inner journey to connect with the Gods/Goddesses, ancestral spirits, and other beings to gain knowledge to assist with their own spiritual growth and the needs of the community. They were the healers and psychologists for their tribe using a practice known as soul retrieval. It is believed that the apple aided the priest or shaman deal with the psychological effects during their sacramental roles in religious rites. This is not new and has been used for centuries in many indigenous tribes.

Apples can provide a practitioner with the means to open a doorway into the mysteries that extend into the depths of the universe. Keeping the spirit safe as it seeks rebirth while gaining an understanding of the nature of eternity, as well as providing longevity. It may also provide an understanding of one's true spiritual self. In Celtic mythology, the silver bough is a branch of apple which bore buds, flowers, and fruit. Accompanied with a magical charm that enabled its possessor to enter the land of the Gods. The golden bough is mistletoe and has a symbiotic relationship with apple trees.

It may also be used as a visionary herb. These experiences are not necessarily accomplished with physical vision. Experiencing them through dreams, trance, divination, or other methods suitable to the practitioner they can assist with a connection with the divine, looking across the abyss for answers to vital questions regarding the self. It may enhance the quality of meditation, helping to sharpen perception.

The early English may have used psychotropic vegetable substances in drinks such as mead, ales, and cider in formal rites to enhance their mystical experience and may also have used this method medically as an anastatic. The term "giddy", meaning dizzy, vertiginous, swooning, from OE giding, (for*gydig), Germanic, guðigaz, ie. "god-y", possessed by a God. This state may well have been reached either by smelling the smoke of the plant directly or mixing it with one of the above suggested alcoholic beverages.

In *Völsunga saga*, Rerir took for himself a wife, but she was unable to bear him children. They prayed fervently to the gods, asking for offspring. It is said that Frigg heard their prayers and conveyed the wish to Óðinn, who in turn gave one of his wish-maidens, the daughter of the giant Hrímnir an apple, telling her to give it to Rerir. The wish maiden assumed the shape of a crow, then dropped the apple onto King Rerir's lap. Sensing its purpose, he visited the queen, and they ate some of the apple. Soon afterward the queen discovered that she was pregnant. King Rerir died a short time later and the queen's pregnancy continued for six years. Recognizing that she herself could not live much longer, she asked that the child be cut from her body. They did as she asked and Völsung appeared already well grown. He kissed his mother who died straight after. He then became King of Hunlan.

Rerir and his wife petitioned the gods for a child, but a gift demands an equal gift in return. They would never get to see their child grow. Their lives were taken as payment for bringing Völsung into the world. There is a clue to the nature of payment Rerir was given the apple by the wish maiden in the form of a crow. Crows have always been symbolic of messengers from the other world and an omen of death in many cultures having associations with underworld deities.

Freyja may also be a symbolic patron of the apple. She is a partner to Óðinn who shared the slain warriors from battle and is a Goddess of fecundity, sexuality and magic as well as being a fierce warrior and a Goddess of violent death. Freyja in the guide of Gullveig brought the magical arts to the Æsir. She and Frigg, (wife of Óðinn), are two faces of the same Goddess. I do not have the space here to elaborate on the subject. This subject and the deeper mysteries connected with them I encourage the reader to explore for themselves.

When the apple is cut into two like the strawberry, the centre resembles the vagina. The ancestors of many older traditions viewed the vagina as the portal to the womb from where life emerges. The gift of life has always been one of the most sacred of experiences known to humankind and has been honoured and celebrated since the beginning of time. This is possibly one of the reasons why the apple was so popular in love magic.

The Divine Matron, Nehalennia, is often depicted with a bushel of apples. She is a Germanic Goddess who is named in numerous votive inscriptions from the third century. Twenty-eight inscriptions come from Domburg on the Dutch island of Walcheren; similar numbers were found in 1971/72 at Colignsplaat on the island of Nood-Beveland; with two others coming from the Colone-Deutz area. (Dictionary of Northern Mythology.

On these votive altars, the Goddess is depicted bearing a basket of fruit, like those from the monuments of the matron cult. The fruit may represent her role as a fertility matron. She is usually accompanied by a dog showing the connection with the underworld and the dead. On vessels, the images were found resting on the bow and even partly on the rudder. Nehalennia name is related to the Latin, (nex, mrvstr), meaning "to kill", which could be evidence of her role as a death Goddess. (Dictionary of Northern Mythology).

Her close connection to ships suggests she is a goddess of seafaring. However, these attributes are also associated with Isis who during the Roman period had been adopted from Egypt losing much of her original role. As the Romans moved north so did the influence of the religion and customs, amalgamating their Gods with those of the lands they invaded or traded with. One important detail should be mentioned here regarding Tacticus's reference in *Germanicus 9*. He had witnessed the Germanic Suebi making sacrifices to Isis. This Germanic Isis in Tacticus has also been associated in various ways with Nerthus. It may be suggested that Nehalennia is a local Germanic Goddess of fertility and seafaring and may have been an earth Goddess like Nerthus.

While Nehalennia's name relates to the Latin, nex, mrvstr), meaning "to Kill, Goddess of death, and/or from the verb, (helan, or "hide) Kauffman's derivation suggests, nēu, which is believed to have a connection with seafaring, but there is also speculation that Nehalennia's name may be interpreted as, "The helpful Goddess coming close" *(A Dictionary of Norse Mythology).*

It is very interesting to note, Njord and Nerthus were considered a divine couple. Their meeting place would be that of coastlines, estuaries, or anywhere the land meets the sea. These places are considered to have deep magical significance. Here where the worlds of land and sea meet, is where a doorway from this world to other worlds may be found. As time moved on and the original symbolism of these patrons had blurred and taken on new symbolism, Goddesses like Nehalennia and Isis shifted from their original roles, with the former, adopting some of the traits which belonged to Njord.

Buckets of golden apples were found in a ship burial in Osberg Norway, while seeds are often found at ancient grave sites. Could this have a connection with the worship of Nehalennia, or did the Germanic people understood the nutritional value of the fruit as well as it being a suitable offering for the Goddess.

There is a suggestion that Hella in her halls also possessed a tree that bore golden apples. These fruits may symbolize both the stress and trauma entering the world of the dead and the healing transformative qualities for which the fruits are well known.

If some are inclined to look at the story of Eve in the biblical Garden of Eden, they may find a different interpretation behind the story than the one that has been given to us over the last two thousand years or so. In the Sumerian myths, Enki offers an apple to the Goddess Uttu. By accepting his gift, she also accepts the offer of becoming his wife. Abella was the god of the apple tree to the Celts. In the Arthurian mysteries, The Isle of Avalon means "The Isle of Apple Trees".

Graves describes apples as a symbol of, "poetic immortality", the letter Ouert. He also writes in, *The White Goddess:*

> The Apple White Goddess is of happier omen than the Blackthorn White Goddess. As introducing the summer....
> It is an axion that that the White Goddess is both lovely and cruel, ugly, and kind. Here again we see the dual nature of this magical fruit.

The Goddess Diana was worshipped in Gaul as Diana Nemeton. This aspect of her was depicted with an apple bough. She was a Goddess of the apple grove. Her festival in Greece was August

13th, (Venus's in Rome), A feast was prepared which included apples that were hanging on the boughs.

The Greeks related the golden apple with the Earth Goddess, Gaea, who presented them to Hera on her marriage to Zeus. They were grown on the tree of life in the garden of Hesperides, the far western realm of the Greek world. The Hesper tribes are the daughters of Atlas and Hesperus.

The apple was the possible cause of the Trojan war where Athena and Aphrodite were in discussion on who was the loveliest. Paris was chosen to make the choice and gave the apple to the Goddess of love Aphrodite. To reward him she gave him Helen. Paris and Helen elope but Helen already married Menelaus who declared war on the Trojans.

There are many myths and stories surrounding the apple. I do not have room for them all here so I will let you discover them yourselves. What they all have in common are the ancient lore connected with this powerful fruit, and the Gods and Goddesses that possess them.

They have been used in divination in a manner of different ways. For example, there is a method in old folklore to reveal the name of a future spouse. The petals of the blossom may be used as a form of divination when cast onto the ground.

On Midsummer's eve, take an apple and peel it, (without breaking the skin). Throw it over the right shoulder and then look. It will give you the initial of the one you will marry. It does work I did it myself, it just took a few years to get there.

Many ancient cultures believed the apple and the apple tree to represent fertility. The Kara-Kirgghiz women who could not conceive would roll under an apple tree. To our ancestors, fertility of the crops, animals, as well as being able to bare and raise children. Was a priority of living in those times mortality rates in children, especially those under five were extremely high.

Even in modern times with better maternity care and with better education on health and nutrition there are still couples who are unable to conceive. Apples, apple juice, or cider would be an excellent offering to Frigg or Frejya for their assistance.

The once popular custom of wassailing the orchard trees, on Christmas Eve, or the Eve of Epiphany, is not quite extinct yet in cider growing regions of England. The word "wasail" was borrowed from the Old Norse salutation ves heill, In Old English, hál wes þú, or wes hál, translation "be in good health". (Oxford English Dictionary. Wassailing involved going from house to house singing and chanting songs offering a drink from the wassail bowl and were given gifts in return. Over the years this custom had transformed into carol singing. Personally, I find the former much more fun.

A further custom was performed over the trees if the orchards to enable a good harvest for the following year. Again, singing and chanting songs were used as part of the rite.

An example of such a ceremony consists of the farmer, with his family and labourer's, going out into the orchard after supper, bearing with them a jug of cider and hot cakes. The latter were placed in the boughs of the oldest, or best bearing trees in the orchard, while the cider was flung over the trees after the farmer had drunk their health in some such fashion as the following:

Here's to thee old apple tree!
Whence though mayest bud, and whined though mayest,
    may'st blow.
Hats full! caps full! Bushel-bushel bags full!
And my pocketsful too! Hazza!

The toast was repeated thrice, with the men and boys often firing guns and pistols, and the women and children shouting.

Roasted apples were usually placed in the pitcher of cider and were thrown at the trees with the liquid. It was believed to be a relic of the heathen sacrifices of Pomona.

Gardeners are encouraged to pour cider on newly turned earth before planting. A libation can also be poured on roots before a ritual. This could be done before cutting a wand from the apple tree. An apple wand may be used in emotional magic and love rites. Spells can be made by using the wood to fashion poppets into figures or carving directly into the wood itself. It is always best to ask the trees permission first before taking any part of it.

It was believed that unicorns lived under apple trees. If approaching an apple orchard on a misty morning, it was believed that if you go quietly and you may observe a raised horn or a horse shape from your peripheral vision.

The mixture of hot spiced ale, wine or cider, with apples and bits of toast floating in it was often called, "lamb's wool", some say from its softness, but the word is really derived from the Irish La mas nbhal, (the feast of the apple gathering), (All Hallow's Eve), which being pronounced somewhat like "Lammas-ool," was corrupted into "lamb's wool," It was usual for each person who partook in the spicy beverage to take out an apple and eat it, wishing good luck to the company.

Another custom connected to the spirit of the apple tree can be found in In Sir James Frazer's *Golden Bough*. A straw figure called "the Great Monard," was placed on the oldest apple tree in the spring. This represented the spirit of the tree. Considered dead in the winter, only to be revived when the blossom appears in the spring. It was believed that the first person who plucks the fruit from the tree, is a representative of the spirit of the tree.

A Samhain altar, (Feast of apples), can be decorated with apples among other items. Apples are considered one of the foods of the dead and a fruit of the soul. They were also buried on this day for those who will be reborn in the spring and have provisions during the cold winter months.

In the English ballad, (*Thomas the Rhymer*), The Fairy Queen warns Thomas not to eat any apples or pears which hung in her garden. For to eat the foods of the dead ensures there will be no return to the world of the living.

Frazer also describes a custom where burning branches were thrown into the apple trees on the first Sunday of Lent to protect the village from fires. Planting a new apple tree was believed to relate to the life of a boy. The health of the tree and its fruit was measured against the health of the boy. There is a similar custom and symbolism in England when planting an oak.

It can be incorporated into rites for unions and weddings, bringing fruitfulness to the couple. As part of the ceremony an apple is cut into half by one partner, giving one of the halves to the other and eating together. This is a charm to ensure happiness, fertility, good fortune and luck.

Apples have long been associated with fertility deities and is a symbol of prosperity, money spells, luck, love, joy, peace, balance, and Apple may also be used in spells and rites to promote one's creativity in all aspects of life to bring an idea into fruition. It is not reserved just for procreation.

There are many ways in which the apple may be used in spells and rites and can be as simple or complex as the individual wishes to make it. The fruit can be offered directly to a patron. Seeds may be planted to create a sacred grove. Bark and seeds can be ground and dried for incense. They can be eaten, and the juice used for a blot instead of mead.

Apples have been used in different preparations for love spells. The blossoms are added to love sachets, brews, incenses, and infused in melted pink wax, strained, and made into candles to burn to attract love.

Great consideration needs to be given before attempting love spells. They should not be used on another without their knowledge. You could spend ten minutes creating a successful love spell and spend ten years trying to release yourself from the relationship because you are incompatible. This can create an unstable and unhappy environment for either or both parties that may inevitably lead to a separation with sadness, bitterness and sometimes tragedy. Any love magic that is performed with a cavalier attitude, manipulation or misused in any way can be met with consequences where the individual wished they had not opened that door.

Medical Use

Apples are versatile, and healthy and make a delicious snack. The health benefits are numerous from one medium, (100g), to an apple a day.

The fun facts about apples are they contain only 52 calories, (based on medium size), and 86% water, Rich in simple sugars like glucose, fructose, and sucrose. They are high in

carbohydrates, but their glycaemic index is low. This means apples have a healthy effect on blood sugar after eating. Despite the popular myth that apples remove plaque, instead, it reduces salivary bacteria which is a similar effect produced by teeth brushing.

A medium apple, (100g) contains 4 grams of daily dietary fibre. Some of these are soluble and insoluble. And are collectively known as pectins. Both are responsible for maintaining a healthy body. The soluble fibres feed the healthy bacteria in the intestines and help with bowel regulation. Insoluble fibre helps move food through the body helping alleviate constipation. Subtle fibres slow the digestion of glucose controlling blood sugar. This can help someone feel full after eating. Soluble fibres are considered effective in preventing cholesterol build-up in the artery's cell walls, lowering incidents of restricted blood flow.

Studies have shown eating 1.9 ounces, (54 grams of apples daily lowers the risk of heart disease and cardiovascular disease. It may also lower strokes by 52%.

Quercetin is a compound that gives plants and their fruits and vegetable their colour. From much research conducted we know different coloured fruits and vegetables have specific and effective health benefits based on their colour.

Catechin is essential to brain and muscle function. It is present in green tea in high quantities and also contains antioxidant effects that help; with weight loss.

Chlorogenic acid that is present in coffee is known to encourage weight loss but may also lower blood pressure. Potassium content is high in these fruits and is essential for heart and kidney health, as well as playing a positive role in other organs when consumed in large amounts.

Apples may cause problems for people with irritable bowel syndrome (IBS) because they contain FODMAPs, fibres which can cause abdominal pain and wind. Thise who have fructose intolerance should avoid the fruit because it may cause issues.

Apples may bolster immunity through its vitamin A and C content. Vitamin C has many health benefits besides. It can strengthen the epithelial barrier against pathogens and can guard against environmental oxidative stress such as pollution and other disease-causing agents carried in the air.

Apples have a cleansing effect on the body's system and are best when consumed in the morning as well as having a freshness that clears the pallet after a meal. In the evening, they have a more laxative action. Sour apples are useful as a diuretic in cystitis and other urinary infections.

Stewed fruit is extremely useful for babies and young children. Useful in gastric ulceration, or ulcerative colitis, diarrhoea, and dysentery. The syrup was believed to be useful for, fainting, palpitations, and melancholy. Cool infusions of the juice were prescribed for fevers and eye infections. While poultices were used for skin infections. An infusion can be made of the fresh raw fruit as a drink to help with rheumatism, pain, and intestinal colic. A cold infusion can help with colds and fever. A tonic made from the bark may be used for gallstones, poor digestion, and intermittent fever. Taken hot it induces perspiration. It has been used for suppressed menstruation. The pure juice, or the juice mixed with olive oil can be a good standby for cuts and abrasions.

Apple cider vinegar can be used in many ways, cleaning dentures, cleaning fruits and vegetables, a tablespoon in the water to make better boiled eggs, flavour soups and sauces, as a hot drink, in the bath, facial toner, dandruff treatment, soothing a sore throat, mouth wash cleaning toothbrushes, whitening teeth, treating acne, getting rid of warts, a natural deodorant, getting rid of fleas, trapping fruit flies, and a weed killer,

Alternative Uses

Apple cider vinegar is often a popular choice as a natural alternative to commercial cleaning agents. This is because of its antibacterial properties. Mix one cup of water with half a cup of apple cider vinegar, and you will have a natural all-purpose cleaner. However, it is worth noting that although vinegars such as apple cider vinegar can kill some bacteria, but not as effective at killing harmful bacteria as commercial cleaning agents. It is a popular ingredient in many steak marinades, giving the meat a nice sweet and sour flavour. Combine it with wine, garlic, soy sauce, onion, and cayenne pepper.

I have used a decent quality apple cider to baked pork chops. Rub the chops in honey and sage and pour the cider over and place in the oven. It has a wonderful flavour.

They are a remarkably diverse fruit. hey can be eaten raw, stewed into sauces, pies, preserves, made into puddings, vinegars, cider, or a fresh fruit drink. Anything you put your imagination to.

Chapter 8

Fennel

OE Finule (*Foeniculum vulgare*)

Fille and Fennel, a most mighty pair!
The wise lord shaped these plants,
while he, holy, hung in the heavens,
he sent them from the seven worlds, seven ages of man,
for wretched and wealthy alike.

Fennel. Large Fennel, Sweet Fennel, Wild Fennel, Family, Appiaceae, Samar, Sweet Fennel.

So, Gladiators fierce and rude,
'Mingled it with their daily food,
And he who battled down subdued,
A wreath of fennel wore.

Henry Wadsworth. Longfellow, (1807–1882),

Growing Fennel

Fennel is grown in Europe, the United States, and most temperate countries. The generic name, Foeniculum, derives from the Latin foenum, referring to the foliar structure. Sow all varieties early in spring in prepared pots or plug module trays, and cover with perlite. A bottom heat of 59–69°F (15–21°C) is suggested to encourage growth. When large enough to handle and after frosts they can be planted in pots or in the garden 20 inches apart. A winter crop can be produced when sown in the autumn. Fennel likes a sunny position in well-drained, loamy, (equal parts sand, silt, and clay), fertile soil. Division of the roots is only possible if the soil is light and sandy. If the soil has a high clay content, mix it with sharp sand.

It is advised not to grow near dill, as cross pollination will reduce seed production, weakening their flavours and the herbs will become cross contaminated. Grown in a hot dry spot produces a sparse clump 4–5 feet high, with thin highly aromatic leaves. In decent garden soil, fennel looks more like a dome of green or purple candy floss. Fennel is an important food source for swallowtail butterfly caterpillars.

The Florence fennel is the only variety grown from seed. Sow in shallow trenches during early summer in rich composted soil, then thin to eight inches apart when they are established. The bulbus roots will be ready by autumn. Give it plenty of water during dry spells. When the root becomes the size of a golf ball, blanch it by drawing some soil around it. After two to three weeks, it becomes the size of a tennis ball and ready to harvest. If grown in pots, do not overwater young plants, they are prone to root rot. Greenfly may occasionally infest the crop; this may be treated with insecticide soap. The young stems and leaves can be picked for sowing and harvested. Dig up Florence fennel bulbs when mature and as required.

There are three main varieties. Varieties. Feoniculum vulgarie Fennel. Garden Fennel. Common Fennel. Green Fennel. A hardy perennial. Height three to seven feet, spread 18 inches. It has many small yellow flowers in umbels during late summer and soft green feathery foliage. Feoniculum vulgare, (Purpurium. Bronze Fennel). Has the same description as above, accept the leaves are an attractive bronze colour. These varieties can be grown in most parts of the northern hemisphere. Feoniculum vulgare, var. dulce. (Florence Fennel), Finochio. Grown as an annual, eight 21/2 to 3 feet. Clusters of small yellow flowers in late summer. Leaves leathery and green. The base develops from a white bulbus. It is a sweet vegetable with a crisp texture and aniseed flavour. This variety can be grown in most environments.

Magical Uses

The classification of elements and signs are varied depending on the source and personal experience with the plant. Most agree that Mercury ruled by Virgo and Gemini would be the dominant element of this herb. However, Fire which is masculine and ruled by Leo and Water the feminine element ruled by the moon in this case fits very well with the androgenous nature of Mercury and its association with the alchemical principle of transmutation. This is another subject that requires more space than I can allow but it is another facet in understanding the plant universe.

In northern traditions, the spirit of fennel was protective on all levels. Fennel was employed in an eleventh century spell to protect cultivated fields. It was mixed with soap, frankincense, salt, and some seed taken from a beggar, the mixture was then rubbed into the ploughshare to ensure safety for the field throughout the coming year. The beggar was given a great contribution for his seed, (a gift always requires a gift to ensure success and prosperity). When it was blended with vervain and dill it is believed to ward off dark magic. Fennel was frequently used as a component in healing powders and potions. It was also employed believing it would encourage longevity, courage, and strength which is probably why it was known as an all-round protector.

Karen Harris in her *Alchemist's Handbook* suggests, the seed, leaf, and essential oil aids in obtaining psychic impressions, owing to its lunar connection, and aiding in interpreting those impressions accordingly, through the power of Mercury. For a protection rite, strew whole seeds in each room, burn in an incense, or make an infusion with the seeds and wash the walls and floors. Burning as an incense or anointing the third eye, clears the mind and aids the memory. The seeds were and can still be thrown at weddings like rice for health and abundance.

Rachel Patterson, in *A Kitchen Witches World of Magical Plants and Herbs*, gives Fennel over to the element of fire and ruled by Mercury, masculine in nature and its ruling signs are Leo, Virgo and Aquarius. She goes on to say it is spicy and powerful, bringing a fresh, cleansing, purifying air. Strong and pungent for a real clear out. It may be used in initiation ceremonies, in an incense or pre ritual bath. This will help clear the path ahead bringing courage and protection while removing the old to make way for the new. Carry in a pouch for confidence and courage. Throw fennel seeds at handfasting to ensure fertility. Fennel can be hung above doorways along with vervain and dill to protect the home. The seeds can be carried on the person in a small cloth bag for the same level of protection. An essential ingredient in purification sachets and healing mixtures.

The Thyrsus which figured in Dionysian ceremonies, was often made of giant fennel stalks with pinecones attached. Wearing a piece in the left shoe is believed to prevent wood ticks from biting your leg. It was also considered to ward off venomous creatures.

In the Stansk region, (Poland), Wreaths for protection and eliminating illness were made of nine different herbs: marjoram, madder, thyme, lovage, savory, basil, fennel, angelica, and hyssop. Girls would throw the wreath on the fire calling loudly "Let go of everything that brings me pain". In the Middle Ages, fennel was grown in the monastery gardens and on the estates of Kazimierz the Great. There was believed to be over two hundred recipes for its use including, a flavouring for bread, an aphrodisiac, and as a tea.

Medical Use

The Romans believed serpents sucked the juice to improve their eyesight. Pliny recommended the herb for "dimness of the human vision". They ate its root, leaf, and seeds in salads, and baked it in bread and cakes. Warriors took fennel to keep in good health, while the ladies consumed it to help against obesity. The Greeks held it very highly and used it as a slimming agent and for many other ailments. The Greek name "marathon" reputably derived from a verb meaning, "to grow thin" is linked to its use as a slimming aid.

The Anglo Saxons used it on fasting days as it calms hunger pangs. In American Puritan communities of recent times, it became known as the meeting seeds. Like dill, the seeds were eaten to relieve hunger during long church services. Culpeper prescribed it as a treatment for poison by snakebite or poisonous mushroom.

The Slavic name for fennel, koper, is derived from the word kopeć which indicated aroma. The seeds were used to relieve gas and was even made into an alcoholic drink. Marcin of Urzędow wrote, "Fennel is known by everyone, it is baked in cakes and bread". It was believed that the root boiled in vinegar would remove a rash or pimples brought on by fevers and half a teaspoon of the ashes of the burnt herb was taken every morning and evening to relieve dizziness. The infusion of the powdered seeds was used as an eye wash and sores.

Fennel Eye Wash

This is very easy to make and is very effective for anyone who suffers from styes or wishes to clear the affected area from any foreign particles like sand or pollen. I have used it myself many times.

Steep one teaspoon of the seeds in a cup of water. Cover for ten minutes and strain. Let it cool before soaking a cotton wool pad in the mixture and wiping it gently across the eye. It can be used to sooth the area by soaking two cotton wool pads, squeeze off extra moisture gently and placed over the eyes for ten minutes.

Make sure hands are washed beforehand. Do not rub the eye harshly or go poking around in there. If pain or irritation persists then get medical help. Damage can easily be done unintentionally.

It can be rubbed into the scalp to encourage hair growth. The seeds relieved colds of the stomach and regulated menstruation as well as acting as a diuretic. The oil distilled from the seed is mainly prescribed for digestive problems and as a mild expectorant, for coughs and respiratory complaints. The essential oil mixed with a carrier oil like peach kernel and rubbed on the stomach area helps relieve discomfort. A chest rub can be made with an essential oil blend by diluting 25 drops of thyme, eucalyptus, and fennel in 25mls of sunflower oil. Shake well and use as a chest rub.

In Chinese medicine a concoction is prescribed for stomach chills, colic, and abdominal pain. A tincture combined with rhubarb or senna can be taken to prevent the symptoms of colic. As well as helping with digestion, the tea can help alleviate constipation. An infusion can be made for gum disorders, loose teeth, Laryngitis, and sore throats. It mya also assist with the symptoms of heartburn.

The root is mainly used for urinary disorders, such as kidney disorders with high uric acid. A sound liver makes real hormonal changes which are the best approach to relieve various symptoms that impact the daily routine. Fennel tea contains phytoestrogens which, according to a study in Italy, improve hormonal balance. Progesterone is the most crucial hormone which makes this herb perfect for decreasing the signs connected with hormonal awkwardness. The estrogenic substances found in fennel tea can greatly affect a woman's hormonal makeup. These phytoestrogens work with the progesterone's to help the impacts of menstruation. Fennel seeds have shown great ability to treat PCOS (polycystic ovary issue), which is a hormonal issue most prevalent in women of reproductive age.

Iron and copper are two basic minerals that develop the generation of red blood cells. Fennel seeds have a decent amount of iron and copper. The tea may increase the rate of red blood cell generation. Potassium is one of the supplements that is found in fennel tea. Potassium assists with pulse control by countering the impacts of sodium, removing unwanted liquids and salts out of the body. It may help aid the reduction of toxic effects from alcohol in the body.

Fennel, also known as finocchio is in the same family as carrots and parsley. An estrogenic herb was used for centuries to promote milk production and is believed to share similar chemical construction to oestrogen on a weaker level. Fennel contains compounds to aid with angina. The Greeks used a tea made from anise and fennel for asthma and other respiratory ailments. They both contain creosol and alpha pinene that loosen bronchial secretions. Fennel seeds can contain 8800 parts per million, (ppm), of alpha pinene whereas anise contains 360ppm.

Fennel is believed to have some impact on body odour. Dr James A. Duke suggests fennel as well as other herbs, (licoricey, thyme, oregano, rosemary, coriander, or fennel), can be used by powdering the herb and rubbing it in the underarm area. This could cause staining to clothes; an alternative is to make a strong tea of the herb and soaking a cloth in it then apply it as a compress for a few minutes.

The tea has an anti-inflammatory phytonutrient called anethole that may have anti-cancer effects. It also has a multicomponent blend containing different cell reinforcements that may help against cancers and may help diminish the risk of growing colon cancer by removing carcinogenic toxins from the colon. Fennel tea may also work with anticancer potential like liver cancer, breast cancer, colorectal cancer, etc. It is beneficial for patients after chemotherapy sessions by helping with disturbances of the stomach chemotherapy causes.

Cosmetic Uses

Like parsley it can be chewed to sweeten breath. Use the seed or leaves for a facial steam and baths for deep cleansing or can be added to face packs. Fennel helps to remove impurities from oily skin, with its deep cleansing and soothing action.

To make a buttermilk and fennel cleansing milk, use 1 cup of buttermilk and two teaspoons of crushed fennel seeds. Gently beat the milk and crushed seed in a double boiler for 30 minutes. Leave to stand and infuse for two hours, strain, bottle and refrigerate, use within one week.

Culinary Uses

Fennel was a favourite herb for stewing in the Middle Ages, fragrant and flavourful with a bonus of being an insect repellent. It was used to flavour food before refrigeration making it edible. The seed can be used in a variety of ways, adding extra flavour to sauces, fish dishes, and bread. Great for winter salads, finely chop the young leaves and sprinkle them over. Lends added flavour to cooked vegetables and add to soups and stuffing's which include oily fish. The bulb of the florence fennel can be sliced or grated raw into salads or sandwiches and can be cooked as a root vegetable.

Chapter 9

Fille (Chervil)

OE Fille (*Chaerophyllum aureum*)

Fille and Fennel, a most mighty pair!
The wise lord shaped these plants,
while he, holy, hung in the heavens,
he sent them from the seven worlds, seven ages of man,
for wretched and wealthy alike.

Fennel and chervil have similar properties in their flavouring with their aniseed notes. In the spell they may be employed together as tour de force. Chervil; Anthriscus cerefolium, anise chervil, British myrrh, sweet cicely, sweet fern, belonging to the species Myrrhis odorata. Native to the Middle East, South Russia, and the Caucuses, it can be grown in warm temperate climates and found growing wild. Belonging to the family Apiaceae, it was almost certainly brought to Britain by the Romans. It is one of the herbs of Lent, believed to have blood cleansing and restorative properties and was eaten on Maundy Thursday. Gerald, the Elizabethan physician who tended the gardens of Lord Burleigh, wrote in his herbal in 1597, 'The leaves of sweet chervil are exceedingly good, wholesome, and pleasant among other salad herbs, giving the taste of anise seed unto the rest'. But is he talking about chervil, (Anthriscus cerefolium), or the species Cicely Sweet, (Myrrhis odorata)?

Growing Chervil

A hardy annual, from the parsley family, (some consider it to be a biennial). Its height is twelve to twenty-four inches and its spread is twelve inches. The flowers are tiny and white and grow in clusters from spring to summer. The leaves are light green and fern like. In late summer it may take on a purple tinge. When young it can easily be confused with cow parsley, (Anthriscus sylvestris). Cow parsley is a perennial and eventually grows much taller and stouter, its large leaves lacking the sweet aroma of chervil. Another variety is, Anthriscus, (cerefolium Crispum), chervil curly leafed. It is a hardy annual and grows like regular chervil, accept the leaf has an inferior flavour.

Scatter on the soil and press in lightly. If it is left to seed, it can provide a crop twice a year. Thin the seedlings to nine to six inches apart, but do not transplant. Medium seeds germinate rapidly as the air and soil temperature rises, provided the seeds are fresh. Young plants are ready for cutting after six to eight weeks of sowing, providing a constant crop if the flower stems are removed. In pots it can suffer from greenfly. Wash off gently with a liquid insecticide soap. Do not blast with a high-pressure hose, it will damage the leaves. In gardens the soil should be light, well drained with plants spaced nine to twelve inches apart. Sow monthly for a continuous crop. Semi-shade is best otherwise it will burst into flower too quickly should the weather become sunny and hot and will be of no use as a culinary herb. For this reason, some gardeners choose to sow in between rows of other herbs and vegetables or under deciduous plants to give them shade.

Harvest the fresh leaves at six to eight weeks old or when four inches tall and can be harvested all year round if they are protected during colder weather. It is not suitable as a kitchen pot plant, it easily loses colour and goes floppy. It should be grown in a large pot on the patio that retains moisture and is in semi shade. Freezing is the best means of preservation; the dried herb does not retain its flavour well. It is good added to vinegar or olive oil.

Chervil is considered one of the herbs mentioned in the healing spell. However, we do not know this for sure as chervil was a late introduction to Britain. Other candidates are sweet cicely, and other species of cowslip, and thyme. In this chapter I will cover chervil, sweet cicely, cowslip, and cow parsley, because some authors are not in agreement on the individual classification of these species and the fold names appear to cover a broader range of plants. However, I will make a case for it being the ninth herb as best I can. I will leave everyone to make up their own minds. Thyme, which is another possibility, I will cover in the next chapter.

Magical Use

An elixir or incense of chervil may be used to put an individual in touch with their, divine spirit, or daemon. In the tarot it may be employed to help the seeker better understand the higher aspects of the card Judgement/Aeon depending on the deck used.

A powerful herb in rituals for the recently departed, after the internment of the remains or corpse to help release themselves from the physical body and guide them to other worlds, or a place of rest until their next incarnation.

Believed to provide longevity in the physical body while helping to connect with their spiritual self and perceive the essence of that which lies beyond death and the nature of being that may be incarnated into a new existence. Not everyone believes in reincarnation, but many do believe in a counterpart that exists beyond the physical and chervil may help them connect in this way.

Chervil is a very versatile herb employed in candle magic, household magic, spells, and amulets. It can be used to bring luck, attract money, strengthening and empowering personal goals, or to empower any working being performed. Generally, this herb brings about change on many different levels. Great consideration needs to be taken before embarking on any working. While focusing on the desired outcome, consider the journey that will have to be taken to reach the destination. What will be lost to reach this goal and is it worth sacrificing and what the impact will be on those around you? The universe gives with one hand but requires payment with the other.

It is a visionary herb and can be employed to extend the vision beyond the physical sense through dreams, divination, or contacting an oracle. As an incense it can improve the quality of visions to enable us to look beyond the abyss to gain wisdom from the divine. Astral temples are important to many traditions across the world. It can be a heaven, a room, a favourite place somewhere, a star, on a planet, or the edge of the universe. Depending on personal preference and magical training, you could be spending a great deal of time there and personalizing it for your own needs. It can be a place to retreat for contemplation, perform rituals when it is not possible to do so on the physical plain, most importantly it is the springboard to the higher realms of wisdom and a place to return to when this journey is done. Chervil, as an incense with all the virtues discussed above, can help the seeker lift their consciousness to take this magnificent journey.

Green Herbs

Chervil is a green herb. These were herbs selected because of having green leaves, nowadays it extends to any herb or spice used to season food which has known magical properties. The kitchen becomes the temple where it is consecrated before use, the implements are the magical tools, and the working space an altar. When the food is seasoned, each herb is blessed, and its deva invoked. These herbs are used to bring about changes for those who consume the food but should not be used without the approval of the guests involved. Anyone who does use the green herbs without consent will be a target for some sharp lessons from the universe.

Culinary Herb

The Polish and other Northern European countries would eat chervil as a green in early spring with sorrel and nettle. It was used in place of parsley and dill for cooking with meats and pickles. Cooked in water and sweetened with honey helped individuals urinate for those who were having difficulty.

The leaf has a parsley flavour with a hint of aniseed and used generously in salads, soups, sauces, vegetables, chicken, white fish, and egg dishes. Add the herb near the end of cooking to preserve flavour. In small quantities it enhances the flavour of other herbs, especially parsley, but also great in a mixture with chives, tarragon, and basil. Stems are chopped and use raw in salads and adds flavour to soups and casseroles. One of the classic fine's herbs, much used in French cuisine with a delicate refined taste. The raw leaves are high in vitamin C, carotene, iron, magnesium, as well as containing other essential minerals. Infuse in tea to stimulate digestion and alleviate circulation disorders., liver complaints, and chronic catarrh.

For cosmetic use the leaf, can be used in an infusion or face mask to cleans skin, to maintain subtleness and helps discourage wrinkles.

Carrot and Chervil Soup

2 oz of butter
2 1/2 cups of carrot chopped
1/3 cup of all-purpose flour
4 cups of chicken stock
salt and black pepper
1 cup chopped chervil
Garnish, cream or plain yoghurt, sprigs of chervil, serves four to six.

Melt the butter in a saucepan and gently sauté the carrots for about five minutes Gently stir in the flour, then add the stock and seasoning. Bring the soup to a boil, cover, and simmer gently for thirty minutes, stirring occasionally. Allow to cool slightly then purée the soup in a blender. Return the soup to the pan with the chopped chervil and slowly bring back to the boil. Do not cook the chervil too long to keep its flavour. Serve hot or chilled with a swirl of cream, or yoghurt, garlic bread, and sprigs of chervil for a garnish.

Chervil Stuffed Trout

2oz butter
2 cups onions finely chopped
2 cups fresh breadcrumbs
1 cup mushrooms finely chopped
Juice and rind of lemon
1 cup chopped chervil
Salt and pepper
4 trout about 8oz or 1 large fish 2–4lb gutted and cleaned

Pre-heat the oven to 350°F, gas mark 4, melt the butter and gently sauté the onions until golden and soft, but not brown and caramelized. Combine the breadcrumbs, mushrooms, lemon rind and juice, with the chervil, and seasonings in a large bowl. Fold the cooked onion into the mix and blend the ingredients well. Divide the stuffing between the trout, spooning it into each cavity. Put a knob of butter onto each fish then wrap individually in a piece of greased tin foil and cook for fifteen minutes. Remove the fish from the oven, open the parcel. It can be broiled, lightly fried, or barbequed for five minutes on each side.

Cicely Sweet (*Myrrhis odorata*)

Also known as Anais, Sweet Myrrh, Roman Plant, Sweet bracken, sweet fern, and switch Apiaceaa. Once cultivated as a pot shrub in Europe it is native to this region and other temperate climates. The Greeks called it seselis or seseli where its name was derived from its sweet flavour. The sixteenth century herbalist, John Gerard, recommended the boiled roots as a pick me up for people who were dull. Culpeper believed the roots could help prevent the plague. There is no information regarding its medical uses having long fallen out of use but was believed to be a tonic for the elderly and teenagers. Seen growing in graveyards in south Wales, it was planted around the headstone to commemorate loved ones. It was rubbed on oak panels to restore the shine.

Osmorhiza longistylis, (Aniseroot) is a plant not in the same species but is used in a similar manner to sweet cicely. Its height eighteen to thirty-five inches. It grows inconspicuous white flowers in loose compound umbels in the summer. The leaves are oval to oblong in groups of three. The whole plant has an aniseed odour. Children would rub the leaves for their liquorice flavour.

Growing Cicely Sweet

A hardy perennial. Height two to three feet and spread two feet or more. The small white flowers appear in umbels from spring to early summer. Sow the seed when ripe in early autumn in prepared seed or plug trays. With the seed being so large, sow only one per plug and cover with compost. Cover the trays with glass and leave outside for the whole winter. The seed requires several months of cold temperatures to germinate. Keep an eye on the compost so it does not dry out. When germination starts, bring the trays into a cold greenhouse. Sowing in spring is successful providing the seed is put into a plastic bag mixed with a small amount of damp sand, refrigerated for four weeks, and then sown in prepared seed or plug trays. When the seed is large enough to manage, (not long after germination), and the frosts are over, transplant to a prepared area in the garden two feet apart.

The tap root may be lifted in spring or autumn. Cut into sections with each with a bud and replanted in prepared plug trays, or in a prepared site at a depth of two inches. Divide in the autumn when the top growth has died down. It is relatively free from pests when grown in pots. One of the first garden herbs to emerge after winter and almost the last to die down.

If the soil is light and well drained, then it could spread rapidly around the garden. Digging it up can be a challenge due to the long tape roots that re-sprout and grow if a little is left behind. If the plant is unwanted during winter, dig up immediately after flowering. Not good to grow in humid areas, it needs a good dormant period during winter to produce its roots and lush foliage.

It does not do well in containers because of the long roots. However, if a container is necessary, use one with plenty of room for the root. Use a soil-based compost mixed with equal parts of fine bark. Place in semi-shade and keep well-watered through the growing season.

Pick the young leaves at any time for fresh use. Collect unripe seeds when green, ripe seeds when dark brown. The foliage and green seed do not dry or freeze well. The ripe seed can be stored in a container in a dry place. Dig up roots for drying in the autumn when the plant has died back.

Cow parsley, Primula veris family Primulaceae, appears to be the species popular when referring to cow parsley. However, as I explained earlier in this book, cow parsley is one plant where authors appear to have a difference in opinion on its identity. I have discovered through my research a handful of species may be of interest includes the common hawthorn, (Crataegus monogyna), not to mention hybridized garden varieties that appear to be included in this category. Because of this it is very difficult to pin down a particular variety that the Galdor was referring to.

There are just as many folk names attached to these plants. I have endeavoured to list as many as I could find. The reader may be able to add one or two of their own based on their own findings. In the text below, I have explained the meaning behind some of these folk names. St Peter's keys, Palsywort, Cowslop, fair bells and keys of heaven. Cowslip primrose, Butter rose, Herb Peter, Paigle, Peggle, Key flower, Fairy cups. Petty Mulleins, Crewel, Bucklet, Palsywort, Plumbrocks, Mayflower, Password, Artetyke, Drelip, Our Lady's Keys, Arthritica, Cuy Lippe. A traditional herb native to northern and central Europe, known as marsh marigold in the US. A legend suggests St Peter let his keys drop when he learned a duplicate set was made. Where they fell, the flowers grew, hence the name keys from heaven.

Growing Cow Parsley

Was considered the first flower of spring and is seen in gardens throughout Europe and the US. The keys, referred to in some of the folk names above are the delicate flowers in yellow, red, or purple in garden varieties. It is a hardy perennial with long oval, wrinkled leaves that are bright green and which spring from a common base. The height and spread are six to eight inches, with a tight cluster of tubular fragrant flowers produced on stout stems in the spring. Oval mid to light green leaves.

Often mistaken for Oxlip (P. elatior), which is a hybrid of cowslip and primrose, (P. vulgaris), of which it has been highly hybridized. Oxlips have large pale-yellow flowers in a one-sided cluster.

Sow the fresh seeds in the autumn on the surface of prepared plug trays, or small pots using standard seed compost.

Cover with perlite or a piece of glass. Place in a cold area or greenhouse. Germination should take around six to eight weeks when covered with glass. Remove the glass immediately when the seeds break through. Winter the plants in a cold frame or greenhouse before planting the following spring. If old seed is sown in winter, then the seed would need to be stratified.

All primula divide easily. Divide established plants early in the autumn by two hand forks back-to-back or dug up in a clump then separate by hand and replant six inches apart. Make sure plants are dug from a cultivated source and are not dug from the wild. They grow best in clumps or drifts rather than singularly.

In containers, all primulas are prone to vine weevil. Water with nematodes, following the manufacturer's instructions in spring and autumn, and when the temperature does not fall below 40°F, 5°C. Use a loam-based compost for container gardens and protect from the mid-day sun. Pick leaves and flowers as required to use when fresh. Dig up the roots of cultivated plants in autumn for drying out.

Culinary Use

Use the young leaves and flowers in salads. It gives a great taste as well as being attractive. The flowers in old recipes were made into tarts, jams, and syrups. It was used extensively in recipes in the seventeenth century. There was an ancient desert comprising of rice, almonds, honey, and crushed flowers. The leaves can be added to meat stuffing.

The flowers can be used to make wine. One gallon of peeps, (yellow petal rings, four pounds of lump sugar, rinds from three lemons all added to a gallon of cold spring water. A cup of fresh yeast is added, then stirred every day for a week. It is then placed in a barrel with the juice of the lemons and left to work. When quiet, it is corked down for eight to nine months after which it is bottled. When ready, the wine should be clear, a pale yellow and has almost the value of a liqueur.

Another old recipe suggests: Boil the water and sugar together, pour over the cowslips which have been beaten, stir well then let them stand covered until almost cold. Add the yeast with the juice of the lemons and rest it for two days. Press out the herbs as quickly as possible, place it in a casket with a hole to allow it to work. When this is done, stopper it for about six weeks and bottle.

To make a syrup: For every three pounds of blossoms use five pints of boiling water. Simmer with sugar until a thick syrup is formed. Use over vanilla ice cream, or an additive for teas.

Medical Use

It contains a fragrant essential oil with two active principles, primulin and saponin. The tea made from flowers is a simple remedy for insomnia and nervous tension and an effective sedative. expectant, relaxes spasms and reduces inflammation, antispasmodic. It is an astringent, and in strong doses a vermifuge and emetic. It is also considered effective in the treatment for bronchitis. Catarrh, dry cough, whooping cough, asthma, arthritis, headache, restlessness, (especially in children). There was an old popular folk belief that, Primrose tea, drunk in the month of May is famous for curing the phrenesie, (old word meaning frenzy) most likely due to its culminative and sedative effects. The roots boiled in ale help deal with ailments of the back and bladder, giddiness, and nervous conditions mentioned above. Not to be used during pregnancy or patients who are sensitive to aspirin or taking anti-coagula drugs, like warfarin. It has been known to cause contact dermatitis.

It is still used by herbalists as a fragrant sedative for banishing headaches. Recommended dosage, one teaspoon of dried chopped leaves and flowers in one cup of boiling water. Cover and let stand for ten minutes. Strain and sweeten with honey if required. Drink one cup a day.

In Poland it is called, Tzebula ogrodowa. Kluczyk learskie, Kluczyki Swietego Piotra, Pierwiosnek. From an ethnographic journal published in 1895, comes a family recipe from Augustów in northeast Poland which gives a recipe for a bouillon to aid bad chests and coughs. In a pot place a chicken, shoulder of veal, handful of cowslip, coltsfoot, and couch grass, a gram of ivy, a few parsley roots, and barley. Cover ingredients completely with water and a tight lid and cook for a few hours until the meat falls off the bone. Strain through a clean cloth and drink morning and night.

In Russia, cowslip is powdered and exported as a vitamin supplement. Clinically used as an extract or powder with other herbs or separately without toxic accumulation as a mild laxative, stomach tonic, stimulant, vitamin builder, and to regenerate the blood.

Externally it may be employed for conditions such as, facial neuralgia, arthritic pain, skin blemishes, sunburn, heat burns, and migraines by making it into a salve or lotion. This is done by extracting the juice from the plant and mixing it with lime seed oil or coconut oil.

It is a feminine herb ruled by the planet Venus, elements earth and water. A little placed under the front porch will stop visitors if you don't want to have company. Carry the herb to preserve youth or restore it when lost. A bunch in the hand will help heal and help find hidden treasure. Placed around the entrances to the home will protect from any harm. In Hoodoo folk tradition, it was also believed that grown in the garden of a home, placed in the pillows of children, steeped in the bath, or sewn into their clothing, would encourage children to mind and respect their parents. A very powerful protector for the home when it is grown near the door, or dried and scattered under the porch, or across the front path, it will keep away unwanted visitors.

Held sacred to Freyja, in her aspect as goddess of love and was used in rituals to honour her. All parts may be used as a spring potpourri. The flower may be used to decorate an altar or for a pre-ritual bath, The whole herb can be transformed into an elixir for priestess for invocations. Although the herb is very sacred to Freyja. it may be used for any goddess associated with love and abundance. It is thought to bring a sense of direction to the practitioner, taking the spirit of the source of the Goddesses energy and help them enter those mysteries that will keep them in her graces. Some believed that following the path to Freyja's mysteries would bring abundance and earthly riches. Cowslip is believed to improve one's attractiveness, increases one's romantic appeal and helps bring about internal changes which stimulates the energy to attract that special partner.

To acquire assistance from the Goddess Freyja in these areas Freyja Norling has an interesting ritual she describes in her Youtube podcast. I have listed it below with one or two additions. Remember to approach her with respect. This deity is not just a Goddess of love, beauty, sexuality, and abundance. She is a war Goddess of blood and violence, an initiatrix and can be brutal and savage. There could be real trouble for those if a cavalier attitude is taken when seeking the Goddess.

How to Connect with Frejya

Take a piece of squared cloth one that is really appealing to you. Select an item that resembles beauty to you personally, and an offering to Freyja as a gift of gratitude and love. Place in the cloth a small item that represents your power, and an item which represents Freyja's presence in your life and a piece of amber. Add flowers to the bundle, cowslips, primroses, and daisies are a good symbolic choice. Wrap it tightly with a ribbon and take it to the nearest ocean, river, forest or anywhere that is special to you in nature. Spend time with some type of devotion to the Goddess. It could be something prepared or purely spontaneous, spoken aloud or silently expressed but let it come from the heart. Either cast the bundle into the water or leave it by the nearest tree thinking about the offering made. When walking away do not look back.

Spells like these are simple and have been performed back into times of old. I have used this method several times myself in the past while living in England.

Sacred to the faerie folk and considered to be lucky bridging a connection between humans and their magical realms. On the yellow disk are five red spots, One on each petal.

On their gold coat spots you see, these be rubies fairy favours, in their freckles lie their favours.

An excellent herb for keeping one's mental focus, while sustaining concentration during ritual work. Believed to help individuals learn the lessons necessary by adjusting positions to further our work. Possesses the energy of abundance allowing the self-rewards for work done well through gifts. Cowslip in water was believed to aid memory for the drinker. This links with ancient myths where a hero was aided by the Gods or other beings to grant them wisdom for victory.

Cow Parsley (*Anthriscus sylvestris*)

The woodland trust gives this description of a species of cow parsley that can be easily confused with those species that are poisonous. If I was to make a choice as to what the ninth herb may have been I would consider this one, or an ancestor of it.

Common names: cow parsley, Queen Anne's lace, (named after a folk tale suggesting the flower bloomed for Queen Ann and her ladies in waiting and looked like the delicate lace on the ladies' garments) mother die, fairy lace, lady's lace, hedge parsley

Fille (Chervil)

Scientific name: Anthriscus sylvestris. Family: Umbellifers. Origin: This plant is native to England and can be found all over Europe and western Asia. It flowers from April to June and can be found in most places with a shaded canopy in woodland, grassland, many urban areas, gardens, and along pathways and on verges. It is a short-lived perennial, tall at around three to five feet with sprays of small, lacey, white flowers. The leaves are divided alternating on the stem. The flowers are umbels, clustering on stalks which come from a common centre. Each flower is around six centimetres and white.

This species should not to be confused with: fool's parsley, (Aethusa cynapium), which bracteoles, underneath the flower head. Upright hedge-parsley, (Torilis japonica), which flowers from July to September, two and a half feet in height smaller than cow parsley. Wild carrot, (Daucus carota), at a distance might look like cow parsley the umbel made up of many florets, has a purple one in the center and its leaves are more like domestic carrots. Hemlock, (Conium maculatum), has similar leaves to cow parsley, but has a distinct spotted stem with purple markings and much bigger, growing to around two meters. **This plant is poisonous and should be left alone.**

It was used in traditional medicines and believed to help treat various ailment, such as stomach and kidney problems, breathing difficulties, coughs and colds and is used as a mosquito repellent.

Chapter 10

Thyme

OE Thyme Odorata (*Thymus vulgaris*)

Just as bees make honey from thyme, the strongest and driest of herbs, so do the wise profit from the most difficult of experiences. Plato

Wild Thyme, (Thymus Serpyllum), is a shrubby herb that grows wild all over the low hills of the Mediterranean region, Asia minor, and Greece. It was introduced to England sometime before the 16th century. Thyme is a genus comprising of around 350 species. Very diverse in appearance and found in many different parts of the world. It may even be found as far away ask Greenland and Western Asia, although the majority grow in the Mediterranean region.

Thymus Vulgaris G. Common thyme, garden thyme. This herb is one of the most popular culinary herbs in use today. Thymus vulgaris. Common, (Garden), Thyme, is an evergreen hardy perennial. Height 12 inches, spread 8 inches. Mauve flowers in summer. Thin, green, aromatic leaves.

Growing Thyme

Thyme is best grown from softwood cuttings, very few are successful propagated from seed. If grown from seed then sow in early spring, spread the seed on the surface of prepared trays or plugs using a mixture of standard and bark compost. A bottom heat of 60–70F, (5–21C) for germination. Do not cover, keep the watering to the absolute minimum as these seeds are prone to getting damp. When the young plants are big enough and after a period of hardening off, plant in the garden late spring early summer 9 to 15 inches apart.

Thyme is easily grown from soft wood cuttings in early spring and summer. The length of the cutting should be two or three inches. Use the same compost formular as above. Protect in winter and replant in spring. Creeping varieties put out ariel roots as they spread which makes them easy to divide in late spring. Stems that are still attached to their parent plant may form roots where they meet a rooting medium. This method of propagation is generally successful because water stress is minimized, and carbohydrate and mineral nutrient levels are high. The development of roots on a stem while the stem is still attached to the parent plant is called layering. A layer is the rooted stem following detachment (removal) from the parent plant. An ideal method for mature plants that are getting woody. To layer, bend the stem down and the target region is buried in the soil in early autumn.

Being aromatic, it normally does not suffer from pests but if the soil is very rich it could be attacked by aphids. Treat with liquid horticultural soap. All varieties will rot if they become too wet in winter. Thymes need to be grown in poor soil, in a well-drained bed to give their best flavour. They are drought loving but need protection from cold winds and hard and wet winters. Trim them after flowering to promote growth and to prevent them from becoming woody. It can be picked all year round.

For preserving, flowers can be dried, or placed in vinegar or oil. The leaves are better cut and dried before flowering. My favourite method with drying any plant is to place them in a brown bag and put them in a dry dark place like an airing cupboard for three to four weeks before placing it in a jar.

Magical Use

This is a gentle herb with a powerful presence. Belonging to the element of water and the sign of Venus as well as Mercury and air. It can be employed in the areas of healing, peace, psychic powers, love, and courage. Burn it in an incense blend or carry in a small pouch to increase health, wellbeing, and good luck. It may also be used to purify and cleanse the home bringing love and encourage a calm, peaceful environment. Thyme may also increase will power and give a person courage. Drinking the tea or added to the bath may help someone to release the past. Place under the pillow to ensure a good night's sleep, bringing peace of mind, and prevent nightmares.

Wearing and inhaling thymes fragrance was believed to help develop psychic powers and allow them to see faeries, especially when a piece is placed under the tongue. In the Middle Ages drinking it in a tea was part of a ritual to gain the same results. Women who wore a sprig in their hair would become irresistible.

The Greeks would use it in their temples for cleansing the space prior to rituals. In spring a cleansing bath of marjoram and thyme can be taken to ensure all sorrow and ills of the past year are driven from the person. Used by the Egyptians as an herb for embalming. Romans used it to purify their rooms, its use probably spread through Europe as the Roman Empire expanded. One of many herbs used in nosegays to purify the odours of disease due to is anti-septic properties. Judges also used it along with rosemary to prevent jail fever.

Used in charms to increase and protect money. An ingredient in Three Jacks and King Oil. Plant thyme in the garden, as it grows so will your money. Another method to increase money is to fold a dollar bill around thyme leaves to make a packet, tie it up and bury in the middle of a crossroads at the full moon. Thyme, mint, and bayberry is a good money protection combination,

A Greene herb, (bringing about change which should not be given magickal power from the chef without your guest's approval). Thyme enhances a relationship already established reminding a couple the reasons they first fell in love, revitalizing the sparks of love and romance in the relationship which has become mired with the daily routines of life.

In days of chivalry, it was customary for ladies to embroider bees hovering over a sprig of thyme on scarves that they presented to the knight. To represent courage and energy. The word Thyme could be derived from the Greek word thumos, meaning courage, and was considered an emblem of bravery. Thyme can be used in spells and potions to increase courage and overcome shyness. It gives a person the power to meet what confronts them and be used to keep a light heart when working hard to achieve their goals.

It was burned to protect the home against dangerous creatures, insects and reptiles and still believed to be used today, especially as an insect repellent.

It may also come from the Greek word Thymos, meaning perfume. It was customary for young women to wear thyme, with mint and lavender, to help them find their true love. It was gathered with marjoram, marigold, and wormwood for love divination on Saint Luke's day October 18th. Take marigold flowers, a sprig of marjoram, thyme, and a little wormwood, dry them before a fire, rub them to powder and sift through a fine sieve. Simmer it over a slow fire and add a small quantity of virgin honey and vinegar. Anoint oneself when it has cooled and before going to bed saying the following lines,

Saint Luke, Saint Luke, be kind to me.
In dream let me my true love see.

Go to sleep and dream of your future partner.

Wild Thyme, (Thymus Serpyllum). The air and aura surrounding thyme is considered to be pure therefore a good plant to have around the house and the garden. One of the furies flowers, tufts of thyme forming one of their favourite playgrounds. The Romans recognized thyme's ability to elevate one's mood dispelling sorrow and melancholy, as well as worn by those who took themselves too seriously to help them lighten up.

In Wales, wild thyme was planted in open graves and sometimes worn at funerals. *The Master Book of Herbalism* informs, "wild thyme we may use to re-establish communication with those friends and relatives who have passed into death". This can be achieved through divination or other methods of communication to seeking council or sending love and blessings. It is one of the herbs used in rites at Hollow's Eve.

Thyme and marjoram were believed to keep milk from spoiling during thunderstorms, by laying the herbs next to the milk. Growing various species of thyme could encourage the divas to become vivacious, (attractively lively and animated), to those with the sensitivity to see, or even sense them. There is much magic to be found in the gardens when thyme is in bloom.

British Smoking Tobacco

Paul Huson in his book *Mastering Herbalism* gives recipes for smoking tobacco blends and a list of aromatic herbs used in tobaccos. He writes that thyme has a pleasant taste as part of an aromatic combination of herbs and can be smoked in a pipe or as a cigarette.

16 parts dried coltsfoot leaves
8 parts eyebright leaves, (Euphrasia Officinalis)
8 parts buckbean leaves
4 parts wood betony leaves
2 parts dried rosemary leaves
1 1/2 parts dried thyme
1-part dried lavender flowers
1 part rose petals, (optional)
1 part chamomile flower optional

Although they do form part of the recipe, the author eliminates the rosemary and chamomile being detracting rather than adding to the flavour. Rub the herbs to a course powder through the fingers or a mesh sieve. Make sure they get a good mixing. He also suggests a milder blend can be made by increasing the proportion of coltsfoot leaves. Any of the aromatics smoking herbs can also be used in accordance with personal taste.

Medical use

The leaves and flowering tops are used in remedies with volatile oils of highly variable composition, mainly thymol, with lesser amounts of carvacrol; flavonoids, (apigenin, luteolin, thymonin, naringenin, others); miscellaneous: lactic acid, caffeic acid, tannins. Regarding volatile oils, English thyme is the strongest, but all varieties can be used.

It contains bactericidal effects of up to 21.3%. It can be used as a deodorant when powdered and rubbed on the body or placed in a cheesecloth bag with a string so it can be hung from a tap in the bath, allowing the essence of the herb to flow into the water as the tap is run., Medical anthropologist, John Heinerman Ph.D., author of *Heinerman's Encyclopaedia of Fruits, Vegetables and Herbs*, suggests drinking thyme tea for headaches. One teaspoon of dried herb per cup of hot water. Use as a compress to ease aching muscles in the neck shoulders and back that can contribute to tension headaches. For a stye, in addition to taking Echinacea and goldenseal, apply concentrated tea directly to the stye with a cotton swab or in a compress. It is rich in thymol, a potent antiseptic, and contains more than a dozen antiseptic compounds. The aromatic oil helps back spasms, make a decoction of the leaf to stimulate circulation. Thymol is a powerful preservative and antibacterial agent, that herbalists use as an antiseptic, a tonic, an aromatic, digestive, and a diaphoretic.

To make a tea for headaches, sore throats coughs and indigestion, infuse one teaspoon of dried leaves and tops, in which a pinch of rosemary may be added, in one covered cup of boiling water for ten minutes. Strain and flavour with honey. Drink as often as required.

To make a poultice mix 2 ounces of chamomile, 2 ounces of lavender, 1 ounce of thyme, and 1 large pinch of ground cloves. Enclose 2 1/2 ounces of the herb mixture in a sachet and soak it in hot water for 2 minutes. Apply to a bruised or swollen area as hot as can be managed without scalding. It has astringent properties that can help reduce the appearance of inflamed skin and reduce pain. The oil is strongly antiseptic and can be applied in a lotion for wounds of the skin.

Used as a gargle for laryngitis and tonsilitis, it eases sore throats and soothes irritable coughs. Excellent cough remedy, producing expectoration and reducing spasms. May be effective in the treatment of bronchitis, whooping cough, and asthma. Make a tea of the herb, allow to cool, and sweeten with honey.

Could be used for infections in the digestive tract which cause diarrhoea. Thyme maybe one of the herbs incorporated with other antimicrobial herbs, as well as essential oil treatments may be especially useful in this area. Thyme like some anti catarrhal herbs work by producing a less viscous mucus secretion which is easier for the body to remove. It has a beneficial effect on the upper and the lower respiratory system, containing a bitter, demulcent, carminative, hepatic, and astringent properties.

Thyme among other herbs produces an expectorant effect and contains volatile oils and digestive bitters, producing antimicrobial effects in the intestines. It contains antispasmodic properties which may reduce muscle spasms throughout the body in general, and/or may work on specific organs and systems. This is done by relaxing the autonomic nervous system, but not necessarily the central nervous system. For this reason, they facilitate physical relaxation of muscles without necessarily causing a sedative effect. The relaxing expectorants have a localized and antispasmodic effect in the respiratory system. Carminatives ease discomfort caused by flatulence. This is related to the volatile oils they contain. These terpene herbs have local anti-inflammatory and anti-spasmodic effects upon the mucous lining and the muscle coasts of the alimentary canal. A cold infusion can be given for recovery from infections and a general tonic. It has also been used as a treatment for menstrual cramps, menstrual regulation, flatulence, colic, headache, and to promote perspiration. The oil is valuable as a local application to neuralgia, headaches, and rheumatic pains.

No side effects or drug interactions have been reported, Preparation and dosage. Tincture dosage is 2 to 4ml 3 times a day, (1:5 in 45%). Infusion, pour 1 cup of boiling water over 2 teaspoons of dried herb and infuse in a covered container for 10 minutes. Commission E recommends 1 to 2g of herb per 1 cup of tea as needed or 1 to 2 fluid extracts one to three times a day.

A dose for infusion is 1 to 3 fluid ounces. To make a tea use equal parts of bilberry leaves, thyme, and strawberry leaves. A tea may be drunk as a hangover cure and can be sweetened with honey.

Household Uses

Flowers are loved by bees and the honey is highly valued. The leaf can make a strong decoction for a household disinfectant. Mix essential oil with alcohol, spray on paper and herbarium specimens for mould protection. The leaves can be used for potpourri. Placed in a draw or wardrobe, it can keep mothballs away.

Cosmetic Use

Beneficial source of anti-aging chemicals. Add a handful of herbs to the bath facial steams, and ointments for spots. It can be used in a face rinse for acne and blemishes, wash the face, infuse equal parts of these herbs in in boiling water for ten minutes and sieve. chamomile, for purifying, yarrow to eliminate toxins, catnip as an antiseptic, lavender also antiseptic and calming, and Thyme as a strong germ killer. Infuse thyme with rosemary as a hair rinse to deter dandruff. The essential oil is as antiseptic in toothpaste and mouthwash. Thyme is used for all skin types.

Culinary Use

Used mostly in savoury dishes but can be used in almost everything. Vegetable juices, fish, cream cheese, meat, poultry, salads, baked fish, seafood, and nearly all soups. Most green vegetables, carrots, tomatoes, onions, and eggplant. sausage, and stuffings.

Conclusion

The Nine Herb Charm will continue to fascinate those who wish to unlock the keys to its mystery and language. Maybe we will never know for certain the precise wording of the literature, but we do know the herbs that are believed to represent the powers being described are potent living entities whether they are used alone, in pairs, or combined together. The more we learn about the ancestral peoples and their methods we may be able to get more of a picture of the deeper meaning behind the works.

Apart from the list of plants I have included above, another suggestion is cockspur grass, barnyard grass, Echinochloe in the family Paniceae. They are widespread and become a nuisance in crops. However, it is cultivated for hay and its seeds are eaten by songbirds, waterfowl, and prairie chickens. It is an outsider for one of the plants but still one to be considered.

In the meantime, we can employ methods of our own to capture the majesty and power of these plants and how to access those hidden worlds that our pre-Christian ancestors probably knew better than we do today.

I hope the information in the book brings the reader closer to their own connection with the plants and the Galdor enabling them to engage and connect on a very personal level.

I always recommend people to try and grow a plant from seed. Watching every stage of development as the tiny stalks come through, the first leaves unfold, the buds begin to unfold and bloom, and the seeds appear ready to produce the next generation. At each stage of its life subtle changes in its chemical composition can be sensed through all of our five senses transporting us to realms of deeper understanding and introducing us to the guides that can assist us in understanding the hidden places of nature.

Bibliography

Albertsson, A. (20011). *Wyrdworking*. Woodbury: Llewellyn Publications.

Andrews, S. (2010). *Herbs of the Northern Shaman*. Arelsford: O Books.

Ann Van Arsdall, Medieval Herbal Remedies: The Old English Herbarium and Anglo-Saxon Medicine, (2010), Routledge.

Association, A. H. (1997). *Botanical Safety Handbook*. American Herbal Products Association.

Beyerl, P. (1998). *A Compendium of Herbal Magick*. Blaine: Phoenix Publishing Inc.

Bonser, Wilfred. (1963). *The Medical Background of Anglo-Saxon England: A Study in History, Psychology, and Folklore*. London: The Wellcome Historical Medical Library, London.

Bremmes, L. (1988). *The Complete Book of Herbs*. New York: Viking Studio Books.

Buddemeyer, J. C. (2018). *Norse Mythology*. Alaska: Chugiak.

Culpeper. (2007). *Culpeper's Complete Herbal*. London: Wordsworth Editions Limited.

Cunningham, S. (2000). *Cunningham's Encyclopedia of Magical Herbs*. Minnesota: Llewellyn Publications.

Dobbie, Elliott Van Kirk. (Ed.) (1942). *The Anglo-Saxon Minor Poems*. Anglo-Saxon Poetic Records, vol. 6. New York: Columbia University Press.

Draco, M (2011). Traditional Witchcraft For The Woods And Forests, Alresford, Moon Books. b

Draco, M. (2002). *Root & Branch*. London: Ignotus Press.

Eshelman, J. A. (2010). *7761/2*. Los Angeles: College of Thelema.

Frazer, S. J. (1951). *The Golden Bough*. New York: Macmillan.

Gloss, J. (2014). *Back to Eden*. Twin Lakes: Lotus Press.

Bibliography

Grattan, J. H. G. and Singer, Charles. (Eds.) (1952). *Anglo-Saxon Magic and Medicine; illustrated specially from the semi-pagan text Lacnunga.* Oxford: Oxford Uni Press.

Graves, Robert. (2013). *The White Goddess.* Farrar, Straus and Giroux.

Grieve, M. M. (1971). *A modern Herbal Volumes 1&2.* Minnesota: Dova Publishing.

Grimm, Jacob. Stallybrass, James Steven. (trans.). (1888) *Teutonic Mythology,* Vol iii. G. Bell & Sons. p1211.

Harrison, K. (2011). *The Herbal Alchemist's Handbook.* San Fransisco: Weiser Books.

Hodorowicz, S. (2020). *Polish Herbs, Flowers & Folk Medicine.* Hippocrene Books: New York.

Hoffman, David, F. A. (2003). *Medical Herbalism.* Toronto: Healing Arts Press.

Huson, P. (2001). *Mastering Herbalism.* Lenban: Madison Books.

Hutchens, A. (1991). *Indian Herbalism of North America.* Massachusetts: Shambhala Publishing.

James A. Duke, P. (1997). *The Green Pharmacy.* New York: Rodale Press.

Kane, C. W. (2017). *Medicinal Plants of the Western Mountain States.* Lincoln Tower Press.

McVicca, J. (2007). *The Complete Herb Bood.* New York: Firefly Books.

Naturelock. (2022, January 14). *Nature lock.com.* Retrieved from Fennel Seeds (Perumjeerakam) Benefits & Fennel Seeds For Weight Loss: https://healthyliving.natureloc.com/fennel-seeds-perumjeerakam-benefits-weight-loss/

Odinsson, E. (2012). *Northern Plant Lore.* www.eoghanodinsson.com

Patterson, R. (2014). *A Kitchen Witches World of Magical Plants and Herbs.* Alresford: Moon Books.

Pollington, S. (2021). *The Early Gods, The Other world of Early England.* Ely: Anglo Saxon Books.

Reaves, W. P. (2018). *Odin's Wife.* www.germanicmythology.com
RH(AHG)., D. B. (2013). *Adaptogens in Medical Healing.* Toronto: Healing Arts Press.
S. Hopkins, J. (2023, December 26). *Mimisbrunnr Info, development in ancient Germanic studies.* Retrieved from Mimisbrunnr Info.: https://www.mimisbrunnr.info/nigon-wyrta-galdor#normalized-and-direct-translations
Simek, R. (2011). *Dictionary of Northern Mythology.* New York: Bohydell & Brewer Ltd.
Storl, W. D. (2012). *The Herbal Lore of Wise Women and Wortcunners.* Berkeley: North Atlantic Books.
The Canons of Edgar, 18, Theodore's Penitential, I. i.4.; and Bede, Eccles. Hist. ii. 13.
The Leechbook of Bald ii
Thistleton Dyer, T. F. (1889). *The Folklore of Plants* D. Appleton and Company. p54.
Trust, T. W. (n.d.). *Cow Parsley.* Retrieved from The Woodland Trust: https://www.woodlandtrust.org.uk/search/?q=cow+parsley&Submit+search=&p=1
Trust, T. W. (n.d.). *Crab Apple.* https://www.woodlandtrust.org.uk/trees-woods-and-wildlife/british-trees/a-z-of-british-trees/crab-apple/
Wright, Valarie, 2007, Heathen Anthology: Volume One, Wise Home Foundation.
Yronwode, C. (2002). *Hoodoo Herbs and Root Magic.* Forestville: The Lucky Mojo Curio Co.

MOON BOOKS
PAGANISM & SHAMANISM

What is Paganism? A religion, a spirituality, an alternative belief system, nature worship? You can find support for all these definitions (and many more) in dictionaries, encyclopedias, and text books of religion, but subscribe to any one and the truth will evade you. Above all Paganism is a creative pursuit, an encounter with reality, an exploration of meaning and an expression of the soul. Druids, Heathens, Wiccans and others, all contribute their insights and literary riches to the Pagan tradition. Moon Books invites you to begin or to deepen your own encounter, right here, right now.

If you have enjoyed this book, why not tell other readers by posting a review on your preferred book site.

Bestsellers from Moon Books
Pagan Portals Series

The Morrigan
Meeting the Great Queens
Morgan Daimler

Ancient and enigmatic, the Morrigan reaches out to us. On shadowed wings and in raven's call, meet the ancient Irish goddess of war, battle, prophecy, death, sovereignty, and magic.
Paperback: 978-1-78279-833-0 ebook: 978-1-78279-834-7

The Awen Alone
Walking the Path of the Solitary Druid
Joanna van der Hoeven

An introductory guide for the solitary Druid, The Awen Alone will accompany you as you explore, and seek out your own place within the natural world.
Paperback: 978-1-78279-547-6 ebook: 978-1-78279-546-9

Moon Magic
Rachel Patterson

An introduction to working with the phases of the Moon, what they are and how to live in harmony with the lunar year and to utilise all the magical powers it provides.
Paperback: 978-1-78279-281-9 ebook: 978-1-78279-282-6

Hekate
A Devotional
Vivienne Moss

Hekate, Queen of Witches and the Shadow-Lands, haunts the pages of this devotional bringing magic and enchantment into your lives.
Paperback: 978-1-78535-161-7 ebook: 978-1-78535-162-4

Bestsellers from Moon Books

Keeping Her Keys
An Introduction to Hekate's Modern Witchcraft
Cyndi Brannen
Blending Hekate, witchcraft and personal development together to create a powerful new magickal perspective.
Paperback: 978-1-78904-075-3 ebook 978-1-78904-076-0

Journey to the Dark Goddess
How to Return to Your Soul
Jane Meredith
Discover the powerful secrets of the Dark Goddess and transform your depression, grief and pain into healing and integration.
Paperback: 978-1-84694-677-6 ebook: 978-1-78099-223-5

Shamanic Reiki
Expanded Ways of Working with Universal Life Force Energy
Llyn Roberts, Robert Levy
Shamanism and Reiki are each powerful ways of healing; together, their power multiplies. Shamanic Reiki introduces techniques to help healers and Reiki practitioners tap ancient healing wisdom.
Paperback: 978-1-84694-037-8 ebook: 978-1-84694-650-9

Southern Cunning
Folkloric Witchcraft in the American South
Aaron Oberon
Modern witchcraft with a Southern flair, this book is a journey through the folklore of the American South and a look at the power these stories hold for modern witches.
Paperback: 978-1-78904-196-5 ebook: 978-1-78904-197-2

Readers of ebooks can buy or view any of these bestsellers by clicking on the live link in the title. Most titles are published in paperback and as an ebook. Paperbacks are available in traditional bookshops. Both print and ebook formats are available online.

Find more titles and sign up to our readers' newsletter
www.collectiveinkbooks.com/paganism

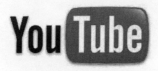

For video content, author interviews and more, please subscribe to our YouTube channel.

MoonBooksPublishing

Follow us on social media for book news, promotions and more:

Facebook: Moon Books

Instagram: @MoonBooksCI

X: @MoonBooksCI

TikTok: @MoonBooksCI